The Physics and Technology of Diagnostic Ultrasound:

A Practitioner's Guide

Dr Robert Gill, PhD

THE PHYSICS AND TECHNOLOGY OF DIAGNOSTIC ULTRASOUND:
A PRACTITIONER'S GUIDE

National Library of Australia Cataloguing-in-Publication entry:

Author:	Gill, Robert.
Title:	The physics and technology of diagnostic ultrasound : a practitioner's guide / by Robert Gill.
ISBN:	9780987292100 (pbk.)
Notes:	Includes index.
Subjects:	Diagnostic ultrasonic imaging.
Dewey Number:	616.07543

Every effort has been made in preparing this book to provide accurate and up-to-date information which is in accord with accepted standards and practice at the time of publication. Nevertheless the author, editors and publishers can make no warranties that the information contained herein is totally free from error, not least because clinical standards are constantly changing through research and regulation. The author, editors and publisher therefore disclaim all liability for direct or consequential damages resulting from the use of the material contained in this book. Readers are strongly advised to pay careful attention to information provided by the manufacturer of any drugs or equipment that they plan to use.

Copyright © 2012 High Frequency Publishing, Sydney, Australia

http://www.ultrasoundbook.net

Foreword

This book has been written to help medical professionals (and others) to develop a sound understanding of the physical and technical principles of diagnostic ultrasound. It is intended for use either in self-guided study or in the context of a formal course or training program. It is assumed that the reader has access to ultrasound equipment and opportunities for scanning patients or volunteer subjects while they are studying from this book.

Inevitably the choice of topics and the depth to which they are covered has been selective. The coverage of the book has been designed to suit the typical university or professional course of study. Practitioners in highly specialised areas such as echocardiography may therefore need to supplement the material here by studying other resources.

The author is well aware that many students of ultrasound find the physics and technology very abstract and challenging. For this reason concepts are introduced throughout the book as they are needed, with each chapter building on the preceding chapters. It is therefore strongly recommended that the chapters be read in the order they are presented.

About the author

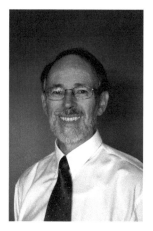

Robert Gill was educated at the University of Sydney (majoring in Science and Electronic Engineering) and at Stanford University, USA, where he graduated with a PhD in 1975. He then returned to Australia and joined the Ultrasonics Institute in Sydney, a highly regarded scientific research organisation which made many pioneering contributions to the development of ultrasound technology.

His primary role was as a researcher in diagnostic ultrasound, with Doppler and non-invasive blood flow measurement being his particular areas of interest. He has published over 70 scientific publications and book chapters, and 150 conference papers on his research and authored 4 international patents.

He developed new techniques for the measurement of blood flow and collaborated with clinicians to explore a number of applications of the technology. Of particular note was his path-breaking work on the measurement of fetal blood flow with Dr William Garrett and his colleagues at the Royal Hospital for Women.

Dr Gill was also active in professional societies. He has been closely involved with the Australasian Society for Ultrasound in Medicine (ASUM) over many years, serving as Councillor, Treasurer, Newsletter Editor and conference and workshop convenor. In 1990-91 he was the President of ASUM. He also represented Australia on the Council of the World Federation for Ultrasound in Medicine and Biology (WFUMB). He was a member of the editorial boards of several international journals.

In 1989 the Ultrasonics Institute was transferred to CSIRO (the Commonwealth Scientific and Industrial Research Organisation, Australia's premier research organisation). Dr Gill gradually moved from research to management and he was the Deputy Chief of the CSIRO Division of Physics when he retired in 2005.

He has always enjoyed teaching and has been involved in postgraduate education throughout his working life. He has taught in seminars, workshops and university and professional courses for the University of Sydney, Queensland University of Technology, Yale University, ASUM (both the DMU and DDU diplomas), ASA (the Australian Sonographers Association), ASMI (the Australian School of Medical Imaging) and RANZCR (the Royal Australian and New Zealand College of Radiologists). Since retirement teaching has become a major activity, leading to the writing of this book.

Acknowledgements

Writing a book, as any author knows, is a ridiculous undertaking. What starts off looking relatively straightforward and manageable ends up taking much longer than it should and causes the author to descend into a state of single-mindedness that comes close to obsession. I am therefore hugely grateful to my wife Margo for her encouragement and tolerance throughout this process. Equally I can never thank her enough for her help in conceptualising and writing the book, proof-reading it (though I hasten to add any errors are my own!) and planning how to make it a reality.

I also owe a great debt of gratitude to my colleagues and friends Roger Gent, Martin Necas, Jill Clarke, Bonita Anderson and Sue Davies. They have generously provided virtually all the ultrasound images in the book, and plenty of valuable advice. My grateful thanks go to Murray Anderson for his design of the book's cover, and for invaluable advice based on his experience in the publishing industry (and as the designer and publisher of his wife Bonita's wonderful echocardiography books).

So many people over the years have helped me to develop my knowledge and love of ultrasound technology. Among others I must thank my colleagues at the former Ultrasonics Institute in Sydney, Australia. Drs George Kossoff and David Robinson taught me much and encouraged me to pursue my interests with enthusiasm, but with an eye to practical outcomes. My colleagues – engineers, physicists, sonographers and technical staff – taught me much of what I know, and it was a delight to work with them, building and putting into clinical operation a variety of research prototype ultrasound machines.

I must also thank my many clinical colleagues. Wise and enthusiastic people such as Drs William Garrett, Tom Reeve and Peter Warren helped to challenge us, spark new ideas and then guide us towards practical applications. Similarly, the many sonographers with whom I had the pleasure of working showed great commitment and enthusiasm, and taught me much of what I know about the practical aspects of sonography.

In my long involvement with the Australasian Society for Ultrasound in Medicine I have been encouraged and stimulated by many who shared my enthusiasm for ultrasound and its advancement. Involvement in workshops, symposia and conferences stimulated my interest in teaching and sharing my knowledge.

Similarly my involvement over many years in university, professional and other courses and training programs has provided me with much pleasure and many challenges. So my final thanks must go to my students past and present, be they doctors, sonographers, engineers or scientists. This book is for them and for the next generation of students.

Rob Gill

Sydney 2012

Contents

Chapter 1

Introduction

Introductory comments

Ultrasound (i.e. high frequency sound) is a very widely used medical imaging modality. It is based on the concept that low levels of ultrasound energy (generally in the form of short pulses) can be transmitted into the body. As it travels through the body the ultrasound interacts with the tissues, creating a series of "echoes".

These echoes can be detected by the machine's probe and processed to produce an image of part of the patient's anatomy. Other forms of processing can produce information about movement (e.g. the flow of blood) using the Doppler effect.

There are a number of reasons why it is essential to have an understanding of both the underlying physics and the technology (i.e. the principles of operation) of ultrasound instruments to be a competent practitioner.

First, ultrasound machines are complex. They contain a mixture of electronic circuits and digital processing, with the trend being towards increasing the level of digitisation. They provide many functions and so there are a large number of user controls. A feature of the industry has been constant technological innovation, with new modes of operation being added on a regular basis.

Secondly, an ultrasound examination is highly interactive. One reason for this is that every patient is different, and that the precise reason for the scan varies from patient to patient. Even something as well defined as a scan of the kidneys will vary depending on the question being addressed. In addition, the details of the examination will be dictated by what is found as the examination progresses.

Thirdly, ultrasound has significant limitations. An important example is the limits to its ability to penetrate deep into the body due to attenuation of the ultrasound energy as it passes through tissues. Equally important is the severe attenuation of ultrasound when it encounters air or bone. This means that the "acoustic window" through which many body regions can be scanned is quite limited.

An extreme example is echocardiology, where windows must be found that allow the ultrasound to pass through to the heart while avoiding the ribs and lungs. The sonographer or sonologist must be aware of these limitations and must be able to optimise both the scanning technique and the equipment settings to minimise their impact.

Fourthly, ultrasound images contain "artifacts", i.e. features in the images that do not accurately reflect the tissues being scanned. These artifacts need to be recognised as such during the examination, and their negative impact minimised. Measurements of structures must be made using correct scanning and measurement technique to minimise the impact of equipment limitations and artifacts on their accuracy.

Taken together, these considerations mean that the sonographer or sonologist must have a deep understanding of ultrasound physics and technology. They must also have a sound understanding of the controls of the machine and how they can be used to optimise the information displayed.

Finally, it is important to recognise that the main priority for the sonographer or sonologist must be to focus on the patient and on the information being displayed. Interaction with the machine's controls and the assessment of technical factors such as artifacts must therefore become intuitive so they do not distract attention from these priorities.

Suggested activities

1. Observe an experienced sonographer or sonologist as they scan.
2. Note how often they interact with the equipment controls and how much (or little) this interaction distracts their focus from the patient and the display.

Physics and mathematics

Physics deals with concepts that help us to understand the physical world – concepts such as mass, force, velocity, temperature and pressure. Most importantly, it also deals with the relationships between these quantities. These relationships are normally expressed using mathematical equations, since any other way of expressing them would be very cumbersome and difficult to use.

You will therefore need to be able to understand equations and what they say about the relationships between quantities. For example, the simple equation $\lambda = c / f$ says that the wavelength of the ultrasound (λ) can be calculated by dividing the ultrasound propagation speed (c) by the ultrasound frequency (f). It also tells us that the wavelength is inversely proportional to frequency; thus, for example, if the frequency was doubled then the wavelength would be halved.

You have very likely forgotten at least some of the mathematics that you will need in studying ultrasound physics. The following section provides a brief review of relevant aspects, including decibel notation, and some examples for you to try.

You are strongly urged to work through it. You will also need to do calculations using the various equations introduced. You will therefore need to have a scientific calculator and be familiar with its use.

Suggested activities

1. Obtain a scientific calculator and practise using it.

   (a) learn to use scientific notation with the calculator, e.g. to enter a number in the form 3.5 x 10^6;

   (b) ensure the angle mode is set to degrees, not radians or gradient;

   (c) practise using functions such as log, sin, cos and $\sin^{-1}$.

2. If you require further assistance with maths, you might like to look at websites designed for this purpose.

Mathematics – a brief review

Equations

An equation is a mathematical statement in which the left and right sides are equal.

It can contain numbers, symbols and functions. Symbols are letters standing for numbers (for example x, y). It is common to use a standard symbol for a particular physical quantity (e.g. f for the ultrasound frequency) but this is purely a convention. Suffixes can be used to allow the same letter to be used for related quantities (e.g. c_1 and c_2 to represent the propagation speed in the first and second tissue).

Examples of functions are trigonometric functions like sine, cosine and tangent (abbreviated sin, cos and tan respectively). Note that $5y$ means the same as $(5 \times y)$, i.e. 5 multiplied by y.

An equation can be rearranged so that you can evaluate one quantity as a function of all the others. This is achieved by adding or subtracting the same amount from both sides or multiplying or dividing each side by the same amount (all of which leave the equation still true). The left and right hand sides can also be interchanged. For example:

$$x = 5y$$

$$\frac{x}{5} = y$$

$$y = \frac{x}{5}$$

and:

$$x = 5y + 6$$

$$(x - 6) = 5y$$

$$\frac{(x - 6)}{5} = y$$

$$y = \frac{(x - 6)}{5}$$

Addition, subtraction, multiplication and division

If several things are added and/or subtracted (or multiplied and/or divided) together, it doesn't matter in which order this is done. For example:

$$a + b - c = a - c + b$$

and

$$\frac{a \times b \times c}{d \times e} = \frac{a \times b}{d} \times \frac{c}{e}$$

An exception is when some of the equation is in brackets – in this case do the part of the calculation inside the brackets first.

Units

Units specify how a particular quantity is measured. Tables 1.1 and 1.2 list the standard physical units for measurements.

Quantity	Units	Abbreviation
mass	kilogram	kg
length	metre	m
time	second	sec or s
electric current	Ampere	A
temperature	degree Celsius	°C

Table 1.1 Units for fundamental quantities.

Quantity	Units	Abbreviation
energy	Joule	J
power	Watts (Joule/sec)	W
intensity	Watts/cm^2	W/cm^2
pressure	Pascal	Pa
velocity	metres per sec	m/sec
frequency	Hertz (cycles/sec)	Hz

Table 1.2 Units for derived quantities.

It is common to use prefixes to modify these units to make them more convenient. For example, length may be measured in metres, centimetres or millimetres (abbreviated m, cm and mm) and time may be measured in seconds, milliseconds or microseconds (sec, msec, μsec).

Table 1.3 defines the meaning of the commonly used prefixes.

Prefix	Abbreviation	Meaning
giga	G	$\times 10^9$
mega	M	$\times 10^6$
kilo	k	$\times 10^3$
centi	c	$\times 10^{-2}$
milli	m	$\times 10^{-3}$
micro	μ	$\times 10^{-6}$

Table 1.3 Common prefixes for units.

Whenever you are making a calculation, make sure the units are consistent (e.g. if one length is in mm and one in cm, convert one of them so they are both in the same units).

You should also look at the units you are using to determine the units that your answer will be in. Write the units after each number or symbol, and multiply and divide units just as if they were numbers.

For example, you are asked to calculate

$$w = \frac{a_p^2}{4 \times \lambda}$$

where a_p and λ are both measured in mm. Then

$$w = \frac{a_p^2 \ [\text{mm}^2]}{4 \times \lambda \ [\text{mm}]}$$

Dividing top and bottom by mm gives

$$w = \frac{a_p^2}{4 \times \lambda} \ [\text{mm}]$$

and so the answer will be in mm.

If you want to change units, once again just write the units as if they were numbers.

For example, if $\lambda = 0.3$ cm and we want to express it in mm instead, we simply replace [cm] with [10 mm] (since 1 cm = 10 mm) and then take the 10 out of the square brackets and multiply by it:

$$\lambda = 0.3 \ [\text{cm}]$$
$$= 0.3 \ [10 \ \text{mm}]$$
$$= 0.3 \times 10 \ [\text{mm}]$$
$$= 3 \ [\text{mm}]$$

Scientific notation

When dealing with very large and very small numbers, it is useful to use scientific notation.

This consists of a number between 1 and 10 multiplied by the appropriate power of 10.

Working with this notation has several advantages. It is easier to read (and get right) and separates the task of keeping track of the powers of 10 from the rest of the calculation.

What do we mean when we talk about "powers of 10"?

You are probably familiar with the convention that 10^2 means (10×10) and 10^3 means ($10 \times 10 \times 10$).

More generally 10^n means 10 multiplied by itself n times, where n could be any number.

Another way of talking about this is to refer to 10^n as "10 raised to the power n".

As an example:

$$\frac{635 \times 0.0072 \times 15}{2870} = \frac{\left(6.35 \times 10^2\right) \times \left(7.2 \times 10^{-3}\right) \times \left(1.5 \times 10^1\right)}{\left(2.87 \times 10^3\right)}$$

$$= \frac{\left(6.35 \times 7.2 \times 1.5\right)}{2.87} \times \frac{\left(10^2 \times 10^{-3} \times 10^1\right)}{10^3}$$

$$= \frac{68.58}{2.87} \times \frac{10^0}{10^3}$$

$$= 23.90 \times 10^{-3}$$

$$= 2.39 \times 10^{-2}$$

Here is another example. The following equation allows us to calculate a particular angle (θ):

$$\sin \theta = \frac{1.22\,\lambda}{a_p}$$

where $\lambda = 0.3$ mm and $a_p = 1.5$ cm. First we will convert λ to cm (using 1 mm = 0.1 cm) to make the units of length consistent:

$$\sin \theta = \frac{1.22 \times 0.3 \,[\text{mm}]}{1.5 \,[\text{cm}]}$$

$$= \frac{1.22 \times 0.3 \,[0.1 \text{ cm}]}{1.5 \,[\text{cm}]}$$

$$= \frac{1.22 \times 0.3 \times 0.1 \,[\text{cm}]}{1.5 \,[\text{cm}]}$$

$$= 0.0244$$

$$= 2.44 \times 10^{-2}$$

Notice that the [cm] units on top and bottom of the equation cancel each other out and the answer therefore is a pure number with no units. This is true of functions such as the sine function. Now we will find what angle has this value for its sine by using the inverse sine ($\sin^{-1}$) function on a calculator. This gives us the final answer:

$$\theta = \sin^{-1}\left(2.44 \times 10^{-2}\right)$$

$$= 1.4°$$

Logarithms

The logarithm is a function related to powers of 10. If

$$x = 10^y$$

then

$$y = \log x$$

Thus the logarithm of a number (in this case the logarithm of x) is the power to which 10 must be raised to get that number. If y is an integer (whole number) this is straightforward:

$$\log 1 = 0$$

$$\log 10 = 1$$

$$\log 100 = 2$$

$$\log 1000 = 3$$

$$\log 0.1 = -1$$

$$\log 0.01 = -2$$

$$\log 0.001 = -3$$

$$\log 10^n = n$$

The idea can also be extended to numbers other than exact powers of 10. For example

$$\log 2 = 0.3$$

$$\log 4 = 0.6$$

$$\log 8 = 0.9$$

$$\log \frac{1}{2} = -0.3$$

$$\log \frac{1}{4} = -0.6$$

$$\log \frac{1}{8} = -0.9$$

Logarithms can be calculated on a scientific calculator using the log function. (Note this is generally indicated by log or $\log_{10}$. It should not be confused with the "natural logarithm" function, written as either ln or $\log_e$, which is irrelevant to decibels.)

Logarithms have a number of useful properties which come directly from properties of powers of 10. Thus the logarithm of a product (i.e. two numbers multiplied together) is simply the sum of their logarithms, and a similar relationship exists for the logarithm of a ratio:

$$\log (a \times b) = \log a + \log b$$

$$\log \frac{a}{b} = \log a - \log b$$

Decibels

The decibel (dB) unit of measurement is based on logarithms. It is always used to express the ratio of two quantities. For example, if the ultrasound power transmitted into the patient is P_1 and the power at a certain depth is P_2 then the attenuation in decibels is calculated as follows:

$$\text{attenuation} = 10 \times \log \frac{P_1}{P_2}$$

In diagnostic ultrasound, decibels are used as the units for attenuation, gain and dynamic range.

P$_1$/P$_2$	dB
1	0 dB
2	3 dB
10	10 dB
100	20 dB
1000	30 dB
0.1	-10 dB
0.01	-20 dB

Table 1.4 Examples of power ratios and their value in decibels.

Some of the advantages that come from using decibels are:

- multiplication and division of numbers becomes addition and subtraction when the numbers are measured in decibels (since decibels are based on logarithms)
- decibels make very large and very small numbers easier to manage
- the calculation of attenuation becomes straight-forward
- the concept of dynamic range would be much more complex if decibels were not used.

Reality checking answers

It is easy to make a mistake when making calculations.

It is therefore strongly recommended that you do "reality checks" whenever you can.

One way to do this is to look at your final answer and see if it seems right. You will learn, for example, that typical ultrasound wavelengths are in the range 0.1 - 1.0 mm. Thus, if you are calculating a wavelength and get an answer of 25 cm you will know that something is wrong and the calculation needs to be checked.

You can also check the accuracy of calculations themselves. As mentioned above, the use of scientific notation separates the task of the numerical calculation from that of keeping track of powers of 10. It is usually possible to do an approximate check of the numerical part of the calculation by mental arithmetic to compare with the answer you have calculated using your calculator.

In the first example in the section on scientific notation above you can approximate the calculation on the second line as $(6 \times 7 \times 2) \div 3$ which gives 28. You can therefore see that the answer from the calculator (23.9) is in the right ballpark.

Exercises*

1. Rearrange $x = 7y$ to give y as a function of x.

2. Rearrange $x - 3 = y + 4$ to give y as a function of x.

3. Rearrange $3x + 5 = 2y - 4$ to give y as a function of x.

4. Rearrange the following to give y as a function of x and z:

$$\frac{(x+5)}{y} = z - 5$$

5. Calculate $3 + 2 - 3$.

6. Calculate $3 \times 2 \div 3$.

7. Calculate:

$$\frac{4 \times (8-3)}{6+2}$$

8. Calculate the following. Simplify it first by dividing top and bottom by the same amount:

$$\frac{5 \times 8 \times 7}{8 \times 3}$$

9. Calculate $(a + b)$ given that $a = 16$ mm and $b = 4$ cm.

10. Calculate $(x^2 + y^2)$ for $x = 5$ m and $y = 20$ cm.

11. Calculate $(x \div y)$ for $x = 1540$ m/sec and $y = 0.2$ mm/sec.

12. Calculate $10^2 \times 10^3$.

13. Calculate $10^{-2} \times 10^3$.

14. Calculate $10^2 \div 10^3$.

15. Write 243,000 in scientific notation.

16. Write 0.000435 in scientific notation.

17. Calculate 2820×0.0032 using scientific notation.

18. Calculate the following using scientific notation:

$$\frac{5780 \times 18.4 \times 0.077}{28.5 \times 0.32}$$

19. Use your calculator's log function to calculate log 20. Verify that this is the same as log 2 + log 10.

20. Calculate $\log (50 \div 25)$. Verify that this is the same as log 50 − log 25.

21. Calculate the sine and cosine of the following angles (using the sin and cos functions of your calculator): 0°, 30°, 45°, 60°, 90°.

22. Calculate the inverse sine and cosine of the following (using the $\sin^{-1}$ and $\cos^{-1}$ functions): 0, 0.5, 0.707, 1.

23. An ultrasound machine has a dynamic range (defined as the ratio of the largest echo to the smallest echo) of 1,380,000. What is the dynamic range expressed in dB?

24. Ultrasound is attenuated by 57 dB in passing through 16 cm of tissue. What is the attenuation expressed as a number?

*Note: The answers to these and other mathematical exercises can be found in the back of the book immediately before the Index.

Chapter 2

Ultrasound interaction with tissue

Ultrasound waves and propagation

Ultrasound is simply very high frequency sound. Audible sound frequencies range from around 20 Hz to 20 kHz, whereas diagnostic ultrasound ranges from 2 MHz to 15 MHz, that is around 1000 times higher in frequency. We will see that these high frequencies are used to provide the best possible image resolution (i.e. ability to image small structures).

Like sound, an ultrasound wave consists of oscillating pressure variations. These are caused by vibration (at the ultrasound frequency) of the ultrasound transducer against the skin surface (see Figure 2.1). When the transducer is moving towards the body it compresses the tissues, causing an increase in pressure ("compression"). When it moves away from the body it decompresses the tissues, causing a decrease in pressure ("rarefaction"). In this way oscillating changes of pressure are created. These pressure variations constitute an ultrasound wave which travels through the tissues at a constant speed.

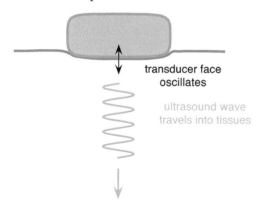

Figure 2.1 Oscillation of the transducer face against the skin creates an ultrasound wave travelling into the tissues.

Since the movement of individual particles and the movement of the energy in the wave are both in the same direction (vertically down into the tissue) the ultrasound wave is called a longitudinal wave.

In this way ultrasound waves differ from ocean waves. They are called transverse waves since the wave travels horizontally along the surface of the ocean but individual particles of water move vertically.

If we were able to focus on a single point in the tissues, we would see the pressure oscillating in time (see Figure 2.2), increasing and decreasing equally above and below the mean pressure in the tissue.

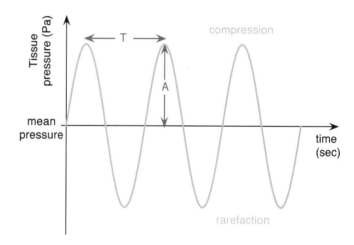

Figure 2.2 Tissue pressure at one point as a function of time. Note the definitions of the period of the wave (T) and its amplitude (A).

Two important parameters are defined in this figure.

The amplitude (A) is the maximum variation of the pressure from its mean value in the tissues. It determines the amount of energy in the ultrasound wave and therefore the level of exposure of the tissues. Useful measures of exposure are the transmitted power (transmitted energy per second) and the intensity at a given point. Tissue exposure will be discussed in more detail in chapter 11.

The period (T) is the time between one cycle and the next. It is related to the ultrasound frequency (f) (i.e. the number of cycles per second) as follows:

$$f = \frac{1}{T}$$

We can also imagine a situation where we could look at the variation of pressure as a function of depth into the tissue at one instant in time. (This is similar to taking a photograph of ocean waves at one instant.) We would find a similar pattern of pressure variations with depth into the tissues, as shown in Figure 2.3.

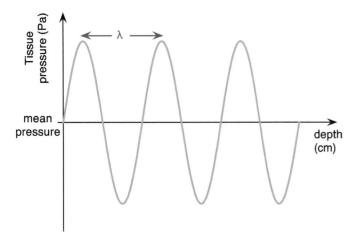

Figure 2.3 Tissue pressure at one instant as a function of depth into the tissues. Note the definition of the wavelength (λ).

This figure shows the definition of a particularly important parameter, the wavelength (λ), which is the physical length of a single cycle (comparable to the distance from the top of one ocean wave to the top of the next one).

Linking these two views – the temporal (i.e. time) variation of the wave in Figure 2.2 and its spatial variation in Figure 2.3 – is the propagation speed of ultrasound in the tissues (conventionally represented by the symbol c). In normal soft tissue it has a value of 1540 m/sec.

We will see in chapter 6 that the propagation speed does vary somewhat, since its exact value in a given tissue is determined by the tissue's density and stiffness and these vary from one tissue to another.

A simple equation describes the relationship between propagation speed, frequency and wavelength:

$$c = f \times \lambda$$

This equation can be rearranged to allow the wavelength for a given frequency to be calculated:

$$\lambda = \frac{c}{f}$$

Table 2.1 lists a number of typical ultrasound frequencies and wavelengths in soft tissue (assuming c = 1540 m/sec).

Notice that for all frequencies the wavelength is less than 1 mm. Also notice that the wavelength becomes smaller as the frequency increases.

It will become clear that the resolution of an ultrasound image is directly related to the wavelength – the smaller the wavelength the better the resolution. Given the inverse relationship between frequency and wavelength this means that:

> *The higher the frequency the better the resolution.*

Unfortunately we will shortly see that it is not possible to keep increasing the frequency to achieve ever better resolution. The physics of ultrasound places a limit on the frequency that can be used in a given clinical situation.

Frequency (MHz)	Wavelength (mm)
2	0.77
3	0.51
5	0.31
8	0.19
10	0.15
15	0.10

Table 2.1 Typical frequencies used in diagnostic ultrasound and the corresponding wavelengths in soft tissue.

Frequency analysis

In this chapter we have implicitly assumed that the ultrasound wave is continuous (i.e. it goes on for ever). This is referred to as "continuous wave" ultrasound. Later we will see that diagnostic ultrasound actually uses short "pulses" of ultrasound (although there is one situation where continuous wave ultrasound is used – "continuous wave Doppler").

A continuous wave is the purest form of oscillation. It is often found in nature, e.g. in the motion of a plucked guitar string or of a clock pendulum. Mathematically it is referred to as a "sinusoidal" wave because it can be described by the sine function. For example, the mathematical expression for the pressure at a point as a function of time (as shown in Figure 2.2) is:

$$\text{pressure} = A \times \sin\left(2\pi f t\right)$$

where f is the frequency of the wave and t is time.

The sinusoidal wave is also useful as the building block for more complex waveforms. Any form of repetitive function can be broken up into the sum of a number of sinusoidal waves of different frequencies.

This process is referred to as "frequency analysis". Thus, for example, a continuous triangular wave can be broken up into the sum of a number of sinusoidal waves of different frequencies, as shown in Figure 2.4.

Note that there are frequency components at the repetition frequency of the wave and at integer multiples of it ("harmonics"). We will return to this concept in chapter 12 when we discuss Harmonic Imaging.

Similarly a pulse (i.e. a wave that lasts just a short time) can be broken up into the sum of many different waves with different frequencies. This will be discussed further in chapter 3.

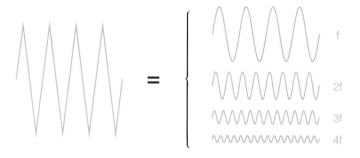

Figure 2.4 A non-sinusoidal waveform (like this triangle waveform) with frequency f can be broken up into the sum of sinusoidal waves of different amplitudes and with frequencies f, 2f, 3f, ... etc.

Suggested activities

1. Look at ripples travelling in water and think about the similarities and differences to ultrasound waves.

2. Calculate the wavelength for ultrasound frequencies of 5 MHz and 10 MHz. Check your answers against Table 2.1.

3. Calculate what frequency would give a wavelength of 0.51 mm and make sure you get the same answer as in the table above.

Attenuation

Diagnostic ultrasound gives useful information precisely because it interacts strongly with soft tissue. In this and the following two sections the major types of interaction will be discussed. These are:

- attenuation
- reflection
- scattering
- refraction

We will start with attenuation.

As an ultrasound wave travels through tissue it becomes progressively weaker. This is referred to as attenuation (see Figure 2.5).

The attenuation is calculated as the ratio of the input ultrasound intensity to the output intensity (I_1/I_2). Since it is a ratio, it is usually measured in decibels (see Mathematics Review in chapter 1 for further discussion of decibels).

It is calculated as follows:

$$\text{attenuation} = \left(10 \times \log \frac{I_1}{I_2} \right) \text{dB}$$

In soft tissue, the primary mechanism causing attenuation is heating of the tissue due to absorption of some of the wave's energy as it passes through.

Why does this happen?

Since tissue is not perfectly elastic there is friction as it moves back and forth in response to the pressure variations in the wave and this means that heat is generated. Energy cannot be created or destroyed and so this process of heating removes energy from the ultrasound wave.

Other factors can contribute to attenuation.

As discussed in the next section, *reflection* and *scattering* from structures in the body cause some of the ultrasound energy to be deflected in other directions. This energy is therefore lost from the wave, resulting in weakening, i.e. attenuation, of the ongoing ultrasound.

If the ultrasound *beam diverges* (due to defocussing or other mechanisms) the energy in the beam is spread over a greater area, and so the intensity of the ultrasound decreases. (Think of a torch being focussed and defocussed and how this affects its intensity).

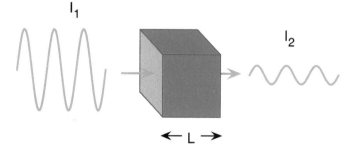

Figure 2.5 Attenuation of ultrasound as it travels through tissue. The amount of attenuation depends on the type of tissue, the frequency and the total distance travelled (L).

The use of decibels makes it particularly easy to calculate the attenuation for a given situation:

$$\text{attenuation in dB} = \alpha \times L \times f$$

where α is the "attenuation coefficient" for the specific tissue involved (in dB/cm/MHz), f is the ultrasound frequency (in MHz) and L is the total distance travelled by the ultrasound (in cm).

For typical soft tissue the attenuation coefficient α is approximately 0.5 dB/cm/MHz.

Thus, for example, transmitted ultrasound with a frequency of 3 MHz travelling to a depth of 20 cm in soft tissue will be attenuated by

$$(0.5 \times 3 \times 20) = 30 \text{ dB}$$

This means the transmitted intensity is reduced by a factor of 1,000 by the time it reaches a depth of 20 cm.

The echo returning from a reflector at this depth will be similarly attenuated by 30 dB as it travels back to the transducer. The total round-path (i.e. there and back) attenuation is therefore 60 dB. This means that the echo coming from 20 cm depth will be 60 dB weaker (i.e. 1,000,000 times lower in intensity) than an echo from a similar reflector at the skin surface.

More generally (see Figure 2.6), the round path attenuation for a depth d (cm) is:

$$\text{round path attenuation in dB} = \alpha \times (2 \times d) \times f$$

since $(2 \times d)$ is the total round path distance travelled by the ultrasound.

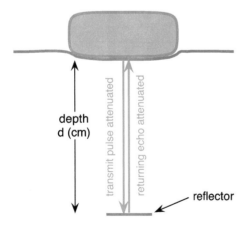

Figure 2.6 As the transmitted pulse travels into the body it is attenuated. The echo from a given structure is then attenuated by an equal amount as it returns to the skin surface and the transducer. The sum of these two attenuation amounts is termed the round-path attenuation.

Returning to the example above, suppose we now decide to use a 6 MHz probe instead, in an attempt to improve image resolution. The round-path attenuation will then be 120 dB, corresponding to a total reduction in intensity by a factor of 1,000,000,000,000! Echoes that have been attenuated this much will be so small that they will be undetectable and will not appear in the image.

> *Attenuation is therefore a fundamental limitation of ultrasound.*

When the round-path attenuation exceeds the maximum that the machine can tolerate, the echoes will be too small to detect and they will not be displayed. The depth (d_{max}) at which this happens (i.e. the depth beyond which the echoes are not detectable) is referred to as the *depth of penetration* (or simply penetration).

For a given machine and clinical situation, the penetration can be calculated as follows.

Since d_{max} is the depth of penetration, we can write:

$$\text{maximum tolerable attenuation} = \alpha \times (2 \times d_{max}) \times f$$
$$= 2 \times \alpha \times (d_{max} \times f) \text{ dB}$$

This will be constant for a given machine and set of operating conditions, depending on factors such as the transmitted power and receiver sensitivity. The attenuation coefficient of the tissue (α) is also constant for a given clinical situation. Thus the bracketed term on the right-hand side of this equation ($d_{max} \times f$) must be constant for a given machine and tissue type.

This last observation (i.e. that the depth of penetration multiplied by the frequency is constant) has profound implications. It tells us that:

> *The depth of penetration is inversely related to the frequency.*

Returning to the example above, we can see that when we double the probe frequency from 3 MHz to 6 MHz we must expect the depth of penetration to halve.

More generally, this relationship means that relatively *low frequencies* (e.g. 3 to 5 MHz) must be used to scan *deep regions* (e.g. in abdominal and obstetric ultrasound) to ensure adequate penetration. For *superficial regions* (e.g. thyroid, breast, peripheral vascular) considerably *higher frequencies* can be used (e.g. 6 to 10 MHz) since less penetration is required.

Note that the use of higher frequencies for scanning superficial areas will yield better image resolution than can be obtained when deeper regions are scanned using lower frequencies. Since we generally want the best possible image resolution, we will therefore:

> *Use the highest frequency compatible with the depth of penetration required.*

Suggested activities

1. Observe which probes are used for different types of examination in your workplace. Notice whether there is a trend to use higher frequencies for more superficial areas.

2. Suppose a given ultrasound machine has a maximum depth of penetration of 20 cm when operating at 4 MHz. Calculate the penetration you would expect at frequencies of 2.5, 3, 5, 7.5, 10 and 15 MHz. Put the results into a table and think about typical clinical applications where you could use each of these frequencies.

Reflection and scattering

Reflection

Reflection and scattering are the two mechanisms that produce echoes and so create the information shown in the ultrasound display.

As with light, the word "reflection" is used to describe the interaction of ultrasound with relatively large and smooth surfaces. (Think of light reflecting from glass.) "Scattering" refers to the interaction of ultrasound with small structures (red blood cells, capillaries, etc) within the tissues. (Think of light scattering from the tiny water droplets in a fog.)

Before we can discuss reflection, we must first introduce the concept of the *acoustic impedance* (sometimes called the characteristic impedance) of a tissue. It is defined as:

$$z = \rho \times c$$

where z is the acoustic impedance, ρ is the density of the tissue (i.e. the weight per unit volume) and c is the ultrasound propagation speed. The units for acoustic impedance are called Rayls.

Acoustic impedance is a useful concept because it is a measure of how the tissue "appears" to the ultrasound.

Two tissues with similar acoustic impedance values will appear similar to the ultrasound, while tissues with very different impedances will look very different. If two tissues happened to have the same value of acoustic impedance they would look identical to the ultrasound.

It is important to realise that tissues may look very similar on ultrasound and yet be totally different histologically. As an example, pus can look very similar in an ultrasound image to soft tissue.

How is this related to reflection?

Consider the three situations shown in Figure 2.7 (a), (b) and (c). It is clear that the amount of energy reflected is determined by the degree to which the acoustic impedances in the two tissues are different.

Mathematically the fraction reflected is given by the following equation, where z_1 and z_2 are the acoustic impedances in the first and second tissue respectively:

$$R = \left(\frac{\text{reflected intensity}}{\text{incident intensity}} \right)$$

$$= \frac{(z_2 - z_1)^2}{(z_2 + z_1)^2}$$

R is called the "reflection coefficient" of the interface (or sometimes the "intensity reflection coefficient"). Since the quantities in brackets are squared, it is easy to show that the reflection coefficient for a given interface will be the same no matter which way the ultrasound is passing through it (i.e. regardless of whether the ultrasound is going from tissue 1 into tissue 2 or vice versa).

Thus, for example, if $R = 0.01$ this means that 1% of the transmitted energy reaching the interface will be reflected and so 99% will be transmitted into the second tissue. It also means that any echoes returning from within the second tissue will lose 1% of their energy due to reflection as they pass through the interface on their way back to the transducer due to reflection from the interface.

It can also be shown mathematically that R is virtually 1.0 when z_1 and z_2 are very different (as in Figure 2.7 (a)) and $R = 0$ when $z_1 = z_2$ (as in Figure 2.7 (b)).

This will be explored in the exercises at the end of this section.

Since energy cannot be created or destroyed, the sum of the reflected and transmitted energies must always be equal to the incident energy.

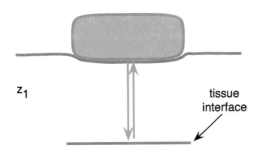

Figure 2.7 (a). Total reflection of the ultrasound energy at an interface between two tissues with a very large acoustic impedance difference (e.g. a soft-tissue - air interface). All of the energy is reflected and none is transmitted into the second tissue. The interface will be seen in the image as a strong linear structure.

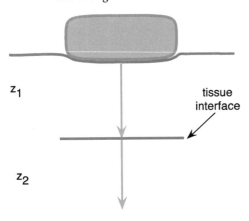

Figure 2.7 (b). Total transmission of the ultrasound energy when the two tissues have identical acoustic impedance (i.e. $z_1 = z_2$). No energy is reflected and so there will be no echo – the interface will not be seen in the ultrasound image.

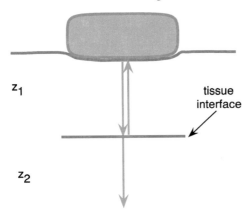

Figure 2.7 (c). Partial reflection of the energy when the two tissues have somewhat different impedances (e.g. a liver tissue - fat interface). A fraction of the energy is reflected and the remainder transmitted. The interface will be seen in the image but it will not be as strong as in the total reflection case.

Taking advantage of this fact, it can be shown mathematically that the "transmission coefficient" T must be given by:

$$T = \left(\frac{\text{transmitted intensity}}{\text{incident intensity}} \right)$$
$$= \frac{\left(4 \times z_1 \times z_2 \right)}{\left(z_2 + z_1 \right)^2}$$

(If you enjoy mathematics, you can check that this is correct.) So far the discussion of reflection has focussed on the special situation where the ultrasound is incident on the interface at right angles (i.e. at an angle of 90° to the interface); this is termed "perpendicular incidence".

What about the more general situation?

When the incidence is not perpendicular, the reflected ultrasound does not travel back to the transducer (see Figure 2.8). As a result the echo from the interface will not be detected and so it will not be seen in the image. (The equations for the reflection and transmission coefficients will also become more complex, but this is beyond the scope of this book.)

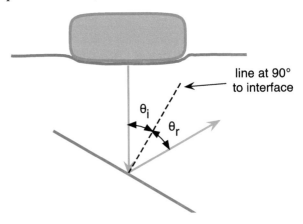

Figure 2.8 Geometry for the reflection of ultrasound from a smooth interface. The broken line is a reference line drawn at right angles to the interface. The "incident angle" θ_i is always equal to the "reflected angle" θ_r. This is the same geometry as for light reflecting from a mirror and hence it is called "specular" (mirror-like) reflection.

Scattering

The word "scattering" describes the interaction of ultrasound with small structures (such as red cells and capillaries) in the tissues (see Figure 2.9). It differs from reflection in two important ways:

- scattered energy is distributed in all directions, whereas reflected ultrasound goes in a single direction;

- the scattered energy is generally much weaker than reflected energy and so the echoes due to scattering are generally displayed in the image as low- to mid-level grey tones.

If you look at a typical ultrasound image you will see that the majority of the echo information in the image comes from scattering from within tissue, not reflection from interfaces between different tissues.

Thus the nature of the scattered echoes and their appearance in the image are very important.

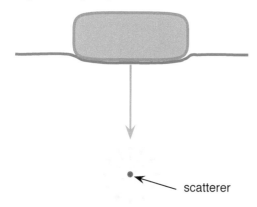

Figure 2.9 Scattered energy is sent in all directions. This means that the appearance of a scatterer is independent of the direction of incidence of the ultrasound. This is different to reflection, which is very dependent on the direction of the incident ultrasound.

You will also notice that scattering produces a random granular echo texture in the image.

To understand why this happens, consider Figure 2.10.

This shows that at each instant the echo signal coming from soft tissue is actually the sum of the echoes from a number of individual scatterers that lie within the ultrasound pulse. Since these scatterers are randomly positioned relative to each other, their echoes will add together randomly. This causes the echo signal received by the transducer to have a random variation in its amplitude.

This phenomenon is termed "speckle" and it gives rise to the "echo texture" that we see in ultrasound images.

> *The size and distribution of echoes in the speckle pattern do not represent the actual location of individual scatterers in the tissue.*

Speckle is a random process that is only indirectly related to the distribution of the scatterers.

To highlight this, consider Figure 2.11. This is an image of an ultrasound "phantom" – a test object made of a gel material containing scatterers and designed to look like liver tissue when scanned. (The strong white echoes come from "point targets" that are used to check measurement accuracy and other aspects of equipment performance; they will be discussed in chapter 10.)

Notice how the echo texture varies with depth. Close to the transducer the texture is quite fine-grained whereas at greater depths it is much coarser. The phantom material, however, is uniform throughout the phantom, highlighting the fact that the speckle does not directly reflect a tissue property.

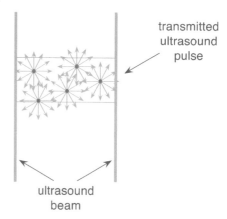

Figure 2.10 At one instant of time the transmitted pulse will "see" a volume of tissue (shown in light blue); the transducer will receive echoes from any scatterers that are within this volume. In soft tissue there will generally be a large number of scatterers within the volume, and the echo signal seen by the transducer will be the sum of the signals from all these scatterers.

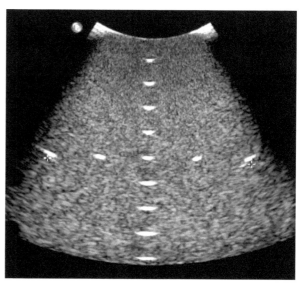

Figure 2.11 Scan of an ultrasound phantom (test object) showing speckle.

Suggested activities

1. Calculate the reflection coefficient at a tissue interface for which $z_1 = 1.5 \times 10^6$ and $z_2 = 1.5 \times 10^4$ (i.e. the two impedance values differ by a factor of 100). Note that the reflection coefficient is almost 1 (or 100%) meaning that virtually all the energy is reflected. Repeat the calculation with z_1 and z_2 interchanged.

2. Calculate the reflection coefficient at a tissue interface for which $z_1 = 1.5 \times 10^6$ and $z_2 = 1.51 \times 10^6$ (i.e. there is a minimal difference between the two impedances). Note that the reflection coefficient is small, which means that very little energy is reflected.

3. Calculate both the reflection coefficient (R) and the transmission coefficient (T) for an interface with $z_1 = 1.5 \times 10^6$ and $z_2 = 1.8 \times 10^6$ (a moderate difference in impedance). Show that ($R + T$) = 1.

4. Carefully examine scans of different anatomical areas and identify which echoes are caused by reflection and which are caused by scattering. Note the differences in appearance of the two types of echo.

5. Scan a region within a liver from two different directions. Carefully compare the speckle patterns – can you see a difference?

Refraction

You are probably familiar with refraction of light – the bending of the light's path as it passes through different materials (as shown in Figures 2.12 and 2.13).

Examples include:

- a prism – a piece of glass with a triangular cross-section, often found in a science laboratory (shown in Figure 2.12),

- the bending of light as it passes from water to air (see Figure 2.13).

Refraction is also the principle on which optical lenses (such as the one in your camera) are based.

Optical refraction occurs whenever light travels from one medium (e.g. air) into another medium that has a different propagation speed for light (e.g. glass or water).

In a similar way, ultrasound is refracted whenever it passes through an interface between tissues with different ultrasound propagation speeds (e.g. from liver tissue to fat).

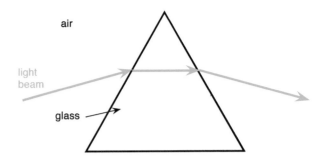

Figure 2.12 As light passes through a prism its direction of travel changes. This is an example of refraction of light.

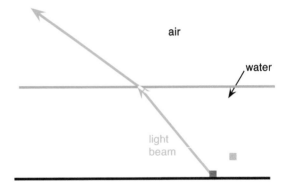

Figure 2.13 Refraction of light coming from an object (darker box) on the bottom of a pool. When a viewer's eye receives the light, the brain processes the information on the assumption that the light has travelled in a straight line (as shown by the broken line), and so it sees the box in the position shown by the lighter box. This is why pools generally look shallower than they really are.

As with reflection, the geometry is determined by measuring the direction of travel of the ultrasound relative to a line drawn at right angles to the interface.

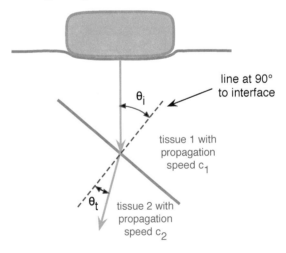

Figure 2.14 Refraction of ultrasound. The direction of travel of the ultrasound is altered as it passes through the interface between tissues with different ultrasound propagation speeds. In this example the propagation speed is lower in the second tissue (i.e. $c_2 < c_1$).

Mathematically the amount of refraction can be determined using Snell's Law:

$$\frac{\sin\theta_i}{c_1} = \frac{\sin\theta_t}{c_2}$$

where θ_i is the incident angle and θ_t is the transmitted angle. It is easy to show that if the difference between the two propagation speeds increases then the difference between the two angles will also increase. It can also be shown that if c_2 is less than c_1 then θ_t will be less than θ_i while if c_2 is larger than c_1 then θ_t will be larger than θ_i (see Figures 2.14 and 2.15).

Comparing Figures 2.15 and 2.16 shows that the difference between θ_i and θ_t also depends on the incident angle θ_i. As the incident angle increases the bending of the beam increases. Conversely (see Figure 2.17) when the incident angle is 0° (i.e. when the ultrasound is perpendicular to the interface) the transmitted angle is also 0° and hence no deflection of the beam occurs, regardless of the propagation speeds.

When the propagation speed is greater in the second medium than in the first (i.e. $c_2 > c_1$, see Figures 2.15 and 2.16) it can be shown that there is a particular value of the incident angle for which the transmitted angle (θ_t) will be 90° (see Figure 2.18).

This value of the incident angle is called the *critical angle*. What is the significance of the critical angle? Since the ultrasound has a transmitted angle of 90° it is barely entering the second tissue – it is just running along the interface between the two tissues. What happens when the incident angle is greater than the critical angle?

In this case ultrasound is not transmitted into the second tissue at all, and instead all the energy is reflected, as shown in Figure 2.19. To repeat this point:

> *If the propagation speed is higher in the second tissue, then a critical angle exists; for incident angles greater than the critical angle, total reflection occurs.*

Thus we have seen that there are two separate mechanisms capable of causing total reflection of ultrasound from an interface between two tissues:

- when there is a very large *difference in the acoustic impedance* of the two tissues, or
- when the propagation speed in the second tissue is higher and the incident angle *exceeds the critical angle*.

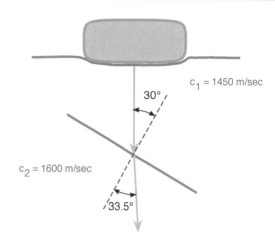

Figure 2.15 Refraction for the situation where c_2 is larger than c_1. The "bending" of the ultrasound is now in the opposite direction to that shown in Figure 2.14. Note that the beam has been "bent" by just 3.5°.

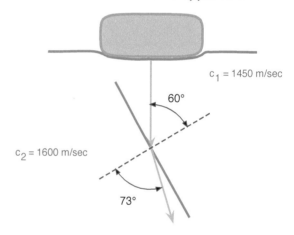

Figure 2.16 An identical situation to that in Figure 2.15 except that the incident angle has increased from 30° to 60°. Note that the effect of refraction is now more pronounced, causing a change of direction of 13°.

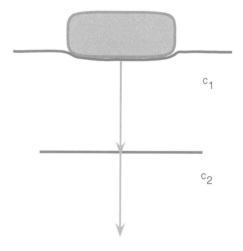

Figure 2.17 With perpendicular incidence (i.e. an incident angle of $\theta_i = 0°$) the beam is not changed in direction at all, regardless of the values of c_1 and c_2.

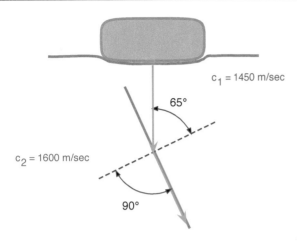

Figure 2.18 When the incident angle is equal to the "critical angle" (65° in this case) the transmitted ultrasound is refracted so that the transmitted angle is 90°.

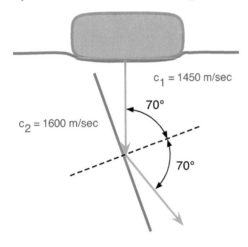

Figure 2.19 When the incident angle exceeds the critical angle, all of the ultrasound energy is reflected from the interface. Notice that the geometry of reflection is then the same as discussed in the previous section, i.e. the reflected angle is equal to the incident angle.

How do we calculate the critical angle?

Recognising that $\theta_t = 90°$ and so $\sin \theta_t = 1.0$, Snell's Law can be written:

$$\frac{\sin \theta_i}{c_1} = \frac{\sin \theta_t}{c_2}$$

$$\frac{\sin \theta_i}{c_1} = \frac{\sin 90°}{c_2}$$

$$\frac{\sin \theta_i}{c_1} = \frac{1}{c_2}$$

$$\sin \theta_i = \frac{c_1}{c_2}$$

As an example, consider the situation shown in Figures 2.15, 2.16 and 2.18 where c_1 = 1450 m/sec (a typical propagation speed for fat) and c_2 = 1600 m/sec (a typical value for muscle). Using the equation above you will find that the critical angle for this tissue interface is 65°, as shown in Figure 2.18.

Summing up, if ultrasound passes through an interface between two tissues with different propagation speeds, the beam path will be bent except for the special case of perpendicular incidence.

The amount of bending increases when the difference in propagation speeds increases and it also increases for large incident angles. In the situation where the propagation speed in the second tissue is higher than in the first, a critical angle exists; when the incident angle is larger than this critical angle, total reflection occurs and no energy is transmitted into the second tissue.

Suggested activities

1. Look for examples of refraction of light in everyday life.

2. Calculate the critical angle for the example above (where c_1 = 1450 m/sec and c_2 = 1600 m/sec) and make sure you get the same answer (i.e. 65°). (Hint: calculate the ratio of the two propagation speeds, then calculate the angle that has this as its sin by using your calculator's inverse sin function (sin⁻¹); this angle will be θ_i.)

Chapter 3

Pulsed ultrasound and imaging

Pulsed ultrasound

Pulse duration and bandwidth

As mentioned in chapter 1, ultrasound imaging makes use of short "pulses" of ultrasound which are transmitted into the body. What do we mean by a pulse of ultrasound, and why do we need to use pulses?

The term pulse refers to ultrasound energy that starts and then stops again shortly afterwards, i.e. a short "burst" of ultrasound energy. Figure 3.1 shows a typical ultrasound pulse. (Remember that the opposite of a pulse is "continuous wave" ultrasound which continues indefinitely.)

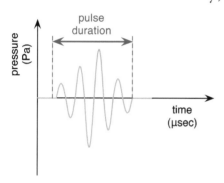

Figure 3.1 A typical transmit pulse, in this case lasting a total of four cycles. Note that the amplitude builds to a maximum and then decreases again. The overall time is referred to as the "pulse duration".

Generally the pulse used for ultrasound imaging is 3 - 5 cycles in length, and so the pulse duration will be 3 - 5 times the period of the ultrasound wave. (Remember, the period is the duration of a single cycle.) For example, suppose the pulse shown in Figure 3.1 has a frequency of 4 MHz. Since the period corresponding to a frequency of 4 MHz is 0.25 μsec and since the pulse is 4 cycles long, the pulse duration is simply (4 × 0.25 μsec) = 1.0 μsec.

When ultrasound is reflected or scattered by structures in the body, echoes will return to the probe and they will produce electrical signals that the machine processes to create the ultrasound image.

Since the *transmit pulse* has the form shown in Figure 3.1, each *echo* will have exactly the same duration and shape (it too will last just a few cycles).

Why is it necessary to use such short pulses of ultrasound? We will see in later chapters that this produces images with good resolution.

> *The shorter the transmit pulse, the better the image resolution.*

As we have just seen, a short transmit pulse can be achieved by (a) transmitting only a few cycles and (b) using as high an ultrasound frequency as possible, since the higher the frequency the shorter the period and so the shorter the total pulse duration will be. This is consistent with the statement in chapter 2 that the higher the frequency the better the resolution.

What are the implications of making the transmit pulse short? To answer this, we need to consider the concept of ultrasound frequency again. As we saw in chapter 2, a sinusoidal continuous wave is the simplest form of ultrasound wave, having a single well-defined frequency, amplitude etc. It is also a useful building block to describe more complex waveforms. Thus we saw that a distorted continuous wave could be broken up into the sum of a number of sinusoidal waves with specific frequencies (f, $2f$, $3f$, ... etc).

The situation with a pulse is somewhat different. Frequency analysis shows that an ultrasound pulse can be broken up into the sum of an infinite number of sinusoidal waves with frequencies spanning a defined frequency range (see Figures 3.2 and 3.3).

While it may seem remarkable that adding an infinite number of continuous waves together can give a pulse that lasts just a short period of time, it is true.

A more convenient way of showing the frequency range is the "frequency spectrum" – a diagram showing the range of frequencies that go to make up the pulse and the amplitude at each frequency – as shown in Figure 3.3.

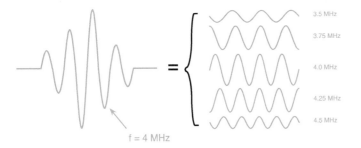

Figure 3.2 A short pulse of 4 MHz ultrasound can be shown mathematically to be the sum of an infinite number of continuous sinusoidal waves with frequencies ranging from 3.5 MHz to 4.5 MHz. Just five of the continuous waves are shown in this diagram for simplicity.

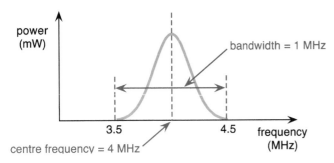

Figure 3.3 The "spectrum" of the pulse in Figure 3.2. Note the definitions of the centre frequency and the bandwidth.

What determines the dimensions of this spectrum? The centre frequency is simply the frequency of oscillation of the pulse (4 MHz in this example); the bandwidth (B) is related to the pulse duration (τ) by a very simple equation:

$$B = \frac{1}{\tau}$$

In this case the pulse duration is 1 μsec and so the bandwidth is 1 MHz. The shape of the spectrum is determined by the overall shape of the transmit pulse (i.e. the way its amplitude increases and decreases).

Notice that the relationship between pulse duration and bandwidth is an inverse one.

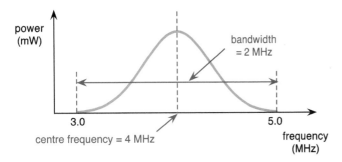

Figure 3.4 Spectrum showing the effect of halving the transmit pulse duration compared with Figure 3.3.

This means that if the pulse gets shorter then the bandwidth becomes larger. In other words, a bigger range of frequencies must be combined together if you want to create a very short pulse. For example, Figure 3.4 shows the spectrum for a 4 MHz pulse just two cycles long. Notice that the centre frequency is still 4 MHz but the bandwidth has doubled because the pulse duration has halved.

Conversely, if the pulse becomes very long, the bandwidth will become small. At the extreme limit, the bandwidth becomes zero for a continuous wave which lasts for ever (i.e. there is no range of frequencies, just a single frequency, as shown in Figure 3.5).

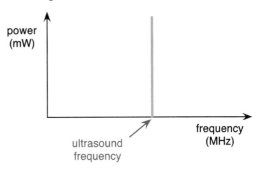

Figure 3.5 Spectrum for a continuous wave signal.

Why does the bandwidth matter? An ultrasound transducer (the active element in the probe) inherently has a limited bandwidth, i.e. it can only process electrical and ultrasound signals within a defined range of frequencies. Since it is difficult for the manufacturers to increase transducer bandwidth, they must ensure that the transmit pulse is designed so that the full range of frequencies that it contains fall within the range that the transducer can process. (If the bandwidth of the transducer is too small, it will force the transmit pulse to become longer.)

Pulse repetition frequency (PRF)

When the ultrasound machine sends a pulse into the body, it travels along a defined pathway (referred to as the ultrasound "beam") and the echoes return to the probe along the same beam, as shown in Figure 3.6. The echoes therefore provide information to the machine about the tissues and structures that are within the beam.

In order to build up an image, the machine must repeat the process of transmitting a pulse and receiving the echoes from the body numerous times, moving the beam so that it passes through a different area of tissue each time. (The movement of the beam is referred to as "scanning"; it will be discussed in more detail in chapter 4.) Thus the machine must produce a series of transmit pulses – usually 100 or more – to produce a single image.

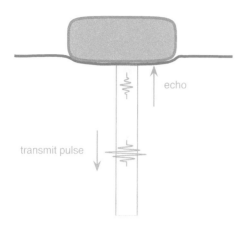

Figure 3.6 The transmit pulse travels into the tissue along a well-defined path or "beam" and the echoes return to the probe along the same path. Thus the echoes provide information about the tissues lying along this path.

Furthermore, the ultrasound machine must create each image in a fraction of a second so that a rapid sequence of images can be created and displayed in the form of a "real-time" (i.e. movie-like) image.

Clearly this means that the machine needs to send out transmit pulses as rapidly as possible. For example, if each image takes 100 transmit pulses to produce and we require an imaging rate of 20 frames per second (i.e. 20 images per second), it is easy to see that the machine must transmit a total of 2000 pulses each second.

The term used to describe the number of transmit pulses each second is the "Pulse Repetition Frequency" (abbreviated *PRF*).

For the machine's electronics, transmitting 2000 pulses per second is no problem. However, we will see in the next section that there is an important consideration (namely the depth of penetration of the ultrasound) that limits the number of pulses that can be transmitted each second.

Suggested activities

1. Consider a 5 MHz transmit pulse with a duration of 1 μsec.

   a) How many cycles are transmitted?

   b) Sketch the spectrum for this pulse.

2. Now consider a 10 MHz pulse with a duration of 0.5 μsec.

   a) Sketch the spectrum for this pulse.

   b) Compare this to your answer for question 1.

   c) Which pulse will give the best image resolution?

3. An L3-7 probe has a bandwidth extending from 3

MHz to 7 MHz (i.e. it can process frequencies in this range). What is the shortest possible pulse duration that can be transmitted using this probe?

Pulse echo principle

We now come to the fundamental concept that underlies diagnostic ultrasound – the pulse echo principle.

Simply put, by carefully measuring the time between the transmission of the transmit pulse and the reception of a given echo, the ultrasound machine can calculate the distance between the probe and the structure that caused that echo. Consider the situation shown in Figure 3.7.

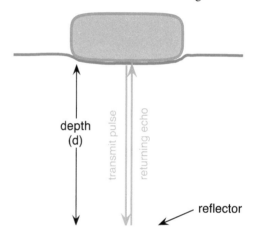

Figure 3.7 Geometry showing the round-path distance travelled by the ultrasound for an echo coming from a reflector at depth d in the tissues.

The total "round-path" distance travelled by the ultrasound (from the probe to the reflector and then from the reflector back to the probe) is simply *(2×d)*. The time taken to travel this distance (and therefore the time delay between the transmit pulse and the echo) is calculated as:

$$t = \frac{\text{round path distance}}{\text{propagation speed}}$$
$$= \frac{(2 \times d)}{c}$$

Rearranging this equation allows us to calculate the depth of the reflector from the delay time as follows:

$$d = \frac{(c \times t)}{2}$$

Thus we see that there is a simple proportional relationship between the arrival time of an echo (*t*) and the depth of the structure causing the echo (*d*).

For the ultrasound machine to use this relationship, it must assume a value for c. It assumes the average propagation speed in soft tissue (1540 m/sec).

As an example, consider a reflector at a depth of 1 cm. Using the above equation gives a delay time of 13 μsec. This is a useful number to remember – for every centimetre of depth the echo delay is 13 μsec. For a reflector at 15 cm depth, for instance, the delay time will be (15 × 13 μsec) = 195 μsec.

Pulse repetition frequency limitations

We saw at the end of the previous section that real-time scanning requires the ultrasound machine to create images as quickly as possible. We will now see how the time taken for ultrasound to travel in the tissues limits the rate of imaging. This occurs because of a fundamental rule that the ultrasound machine must obey (see Figure 3.8):

> *The machine must not transmit again until all detectable echoes caused by the previous transmit pulse have been received.*

If the machine violates this rule, echoes from the new transmit pulse will overlap with the echoes from the previous pulse and an artifact known as "range ambiguity" will occur. We will consider this in more detail in chapter 8.

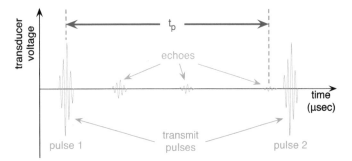

Figure 3.8 The voltage seen on the transducer as a function of time. The first transmit pulse is followed by a series of echoes (only three are shown here for simplicity), diminishing in amplitude until they become undetectable. The time from the transmit pulse to the last detectable echo is t_p. The next pulse can only be transmitted after this time.

Now consider a probe which penetrates to a depth P. (Reminder: this means that echoes from structures at depths greater than P are not detectable.) Since we know the relationship between depth and echo arrival time, we can calculate when the last detectable echo will be received.

The time delay between the transmit pulse and the last detectable echo (t_p) is given by:

$$t_p = \frac{(2 \times P)}{c}$$

Given the rule cited above, this will be the shortest allowable time between one transmit pulse and the next. It follows therefore that the maximum number of transmit pulses per second will be the reciprocal of this time:

$$\text{maximum PRF} = \frac{c}{(2 \times P)}$$

Remember that "Pulse Repetition Frequency" (PRF) means the total number of pulses transmitted each second.

Since the machine generally strives to produce as many images each second as possible, it will make an estimate of the depth of penetration P (taking into account the ultrasound frequency being used) and then it will use the maximum PRF consistent with that depth of penetration.

The above relationship between the maximum allowable PRF and the depth of penetration is an inverse one. Thus, if the depth of penetration is small (e.g. in a carotid artery scan) a high PRF can be used and so the frame rate will also be high. Conversely, we can see that having a large depth of penetration (as generally required in an abdominal scan, for example) will force the machine to use a relatively low PRF and so decrease the rate of imaging.

Frame rate limitations

Now that we know how to calculate the maximum allowable PRF that the machine can use, it is relatively easy to calculate the maximum possible imaging rate. Note that the number of images created each second is termed the "Frame Rate" (abbreviated FR).

If the machine requires N transmit pulses to create each image, it is easy to see that the total number of pulses required each second is simply ($N \times FR$). Since the total number of transmit pulses available each second is by definition the PRF, we have:

$$N \times FR = PRF$$

and therefore

$$FR = \frac{PRF}{N}$$

The frame rate is directly proportional to the PRF and inversely proportional to the number of pulses required to produce each image.

Now we can introduce the previously derived equation relating the maximum allowable *PRF* and the depth of penetration (*P*). This gives us the following relationship between the maximum possible frame rate, the depth of penetration and the number of transmit pulses required to create each image:

$$FR = \frac{c}{(2 \times P \times N)}$$

This is more commonly rearranged and written as follows:

$$(FR \times P \times N) = \frac{c}{2}$$

Assuming that the frame rate (*FR*) is expressed in frames/sec and the penetration (*P*) is measured in cm, then we can substitute the usual value for the propagation speed in soft tissue, converting it to cm/sec for consistency (i.e. *c* = 1540 m/sec = 154,000 cm/sec). This gives:

$$(FR \times P \times N) = 77,000 \text{ cm/sec}$$

The product of the three quantities on the left of this equation is thus limited by a physical constant which we cannot alter (the propagation speed divided by two). Therefore, if we want to increase any one of these three quantities (e.g. frame rate), one or both of the other two must be decreased to compensate.

For example, consider an abdominal scan where we require a depth of penetration of 25 cm. Suppose that the ultrasound machine needs a total of 100 transmit pulses to create each image. Then the above equation tells us that the maximum possible frame rate is 30 frames per second.

While this is quite adequate for most applications, there are some clinical areas (such as echocardiography) where we may want to increase the frame rate above this value. Suppose we wanted a frame rate of 60 frames per second, but still required the 25 cm depth of penetration. Then the equation above tells us that the number of pulses for each image would need to drop to 50.

In echocardiography it is often possible to achieve this by narrowing the field of view of the transducer so that less pulses are needed to create each image.

We will revisit the issue of frame rate under the heading Temporal Resolution in chapter 10. In particular, we will take account of the fact that many machines are able to produce several beams at once. This "multiple beamforming" capability speeds up the acquisition of echo information, increasing the frame rate significantly.

SUMMARY

This story has become complex, so let us recapitulate:

- *To create an image, the machine transmits ultrasound pulses and collects the echoes that come back from structures within the tissues.*

- *The time taken for each pulse to travel into the tissue and for the echoes to return depends on the depth of penetration (P) of the ultrasound; the greater the depth the longer it takes for the echoes to return.*

- *The machine must transmit a number of pulses (N, typically 100 or so) to create each image.*

- *Thus the overall time taken to produce one image will be determined by both P and N.*

- *The number of images that can be produced each second (i.e. the frame rate FR) is therefore also a function of both P and N.*

- *High frame rates can be achieved if the depth of penetration is small and/or if a relatively small number of transmit pulses are needed to create each image.*

Suggested activities

1. Consider a 10 MHz probe used for breast scanning. Suppose that it has a depth of penetration of 8 cm.

   (a) Calculate the delay between the transmit pulse and the last detectable echo.

   (b) Suppose that the machine requires 200 transmit pulses to create an image. Calculate how long it takes to create an image.

   (c) Using the answer to (b), calculate the frame rate (i.e. how many images will be created each second).

   (d) Check that $(FR \times P \times N) = 77,000$. Don't be concerned if you don't get exactly 77,000 – this will be due to rounding errors.

2. Note the actual frame rate at which a clinical ultrasound machine operates and whether the frame rate changes when you switch from a low frequency probe to a high frequency probe. Consider whether the differences that you observe are consistent with the above discussion.

Principles of image formation

The previous sections have described the basis of ultrasound imaging:

- The machine's probe transmits a short pulse of ultrasound into the patient's body.
- This pulse travels along a defined pathway referred to as the ultrasound "beam".
- Structures within the beam cause some of the transmitted energy to be reflected and scattered.
- Some of the reflected and scattered energy travels back along the beam to the probe, where it is detected and converted into an electrical signal.

The signal due to an individual structure is referred to as an "echo". As we have seen, by measuring the exact arrival time of an echo the machine can calculate the distance from the probe to the structure that caused it. The machine also knows the position of the beam relative to the probe, and so it is able to define relatively accurately where the structure is within the ultrasound image. This allows it to place a point in the image to represent the structure, as shown in Figure 3.9.

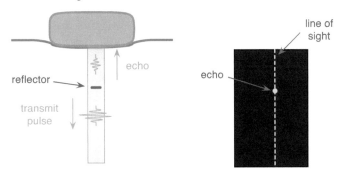

Figure 3.9 (Left) Reflected ultrasound returning to the probe will give rise to an echo signal. (Right) On the machine's display the echo will be displayed as a dot. Note that it is placed in the image (the black rectangle) at the correct depth and on a "line of sight" that corresponds to the centre-line of the beam.

The brightness of the dot is determined by the intensity of the echo. A weak echo will be shown as a dark grey, a moderate intensity echo as a mid-grey and a strong echo as white. Black is shown when no echoes are detected.

Three standard types of probe are used with ultrasound machines (see Figure 3.10):

- linear arrays;
- curved arrays (sometimes called "curvilinear" or "convex" arrays);
- phased arrays.

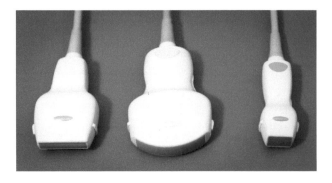

Figure 3.10 (left to right) Typical linear, curved and phased array probes.

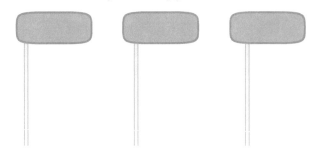

Figure 3.11 (a) In a linear array the beam is stepped from left to right for successive transmit pulses (only the first three beam positions are shown).

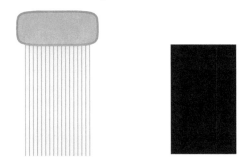

Figure 3.11 (b) As the beam moves from one end of the probe to the other it sweeps out a rectangular field of view and so the image (black) is rectangular.

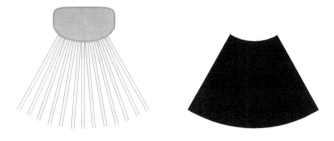

Figure 3.12 A curved array is similar to a linear array. However, due to the curvature of the probe the lines of sight are not parallel, but instead sweep out a radial path. This type of probe therefore provides a significantly wider field of view than the linear array.

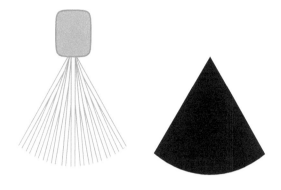

Figure 3.13 Phased array. The point of origin of the beam remains fixed. It is scanned by steering it in a series of different directions. The resulting image provides a good field of view at depth, but virtually no information about superficial tissues.

As we will see shortly, the word "array" refers to the fact that the transducer (the active element in the probe) is sliced into a large number of identical transducer "elements" to facilitate electronic focussing and scanning of the ultrasound beam.

Figures 3.11, 3.12 and 3.13 illustrate the scan patterns and image shape for these three probe types. Why are different types of probe used in different clinical applications? The answer lies in their relative strengths and limitations. These relate to considerations such as the physical size of the probe (often called its "footprint"), the available "acoustic window" into the patient (i.e. the area in the superficial tissues through which ultrasound can travel) and the shape and elasticity of the skin where the probe is to be placed.

In some areas (e.g. transthoracic echocardiography, where the ultrasound must travel between ribs and must avoid the lungs) the acoustic window is extremely limited. In other areas (e.g. late pregnancy scans) the acoustic window is large and therefore not such a concern.

In summary:

Linear array: ideal for relatively flat surfaces such as the neck and limbs; however, the field of view is limited by the probe dimensions.

Curved array: widely useful, probably the standard probe in most clinical areas; the field of view diverges with depth, so it is not so limited by probe size or the acoustic window; the degree of divergence depends on the degree of curvature of the probe and so it can be tailored to suit a given clinical application.

Phased array: the dominant probe type in echocardiography; compact, easily manipulated and able to make use of a very small acoustic window; major limitation is the lack of detail close to the probe.

Two other types of probe are available for use in specific situations, namely invasive and 3D probes.

Invasive probes include transvaginal (see Figure 3.14), transrectal and transoesophageal. As with standard probes they use array technology to focus and scan the beam.

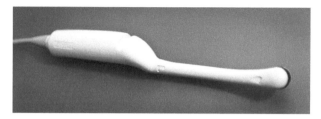

Figure 3.14 Transvaginal probe.

An advantage often claimed for ultrasound is that it is non-invasive, so why are invasive probes used? There are two reasons. First, some areas are virtually impossible to reach with ultrasound from the skin surface because of intervening gas and bone. An invasive probe can get very close to the region of interest (ovaries, prostate, aortic outflow tract etc) and so avoid the problems relating to overlying tissues.

Secondly, the fact that the probe is close to the tissues of interest means that a higher frequency can be used and so the image resolution is improved over what could be achieved with standard (non-invasive) scanning.

As discussed in chapter 12, 3D imaging places an extra requirement on the probe. The scan plane must be swept through the patient's tissues in order to acquire echo information from a three dimensional volume. Historically this has been achieved by moving the transducer, either manually or mechanically. More recently, however, it has become possible to achieve the same thing electronically using "matrix" transducers, which will be discussed more fully in chapter 4.

A, B and M mode

The technique used to produce the standard ultrasound image is referred to as "B-mode" (Brightness mode) imaging. Note that it produces a two-dimensional image of the patient's anatomy. Two other imaging modes are used in specific clinical areas, both of them one-dimensional.

"M-mode" (Motion mode) is widely use in echocardiography to provide detailed information regarding the movements of the heart walls and valves. To produce an M-mode display, the machine keeps the ultrasound beam in a fixed position and repeatedly transmits and receives along this beam. The display of the echoes is swept slowly from left to right on the screen over a period of several seconds.

Structures that are stationary relative to the probe (e.g. the chest wall) will be displayed at a constant depth and therefore as horizontal lines, while structures that move towards and away from the probe (e.g. the heart walls) will move up and down the screen and so the display will document their position as a function of time, as shown in Figure 3.15.

The M-mode display thus provides information about the amount of movement of individual structures, the speed at which they move and their acceleration.

It also shows the relative position of structures and how that changes with time (e.g. the maximum and minimum diameters of a heart chamber, or the movement of two valve leaflets as the valve opens and closes). Often an ECG trace is also shown on the screen to provide a timing reference.

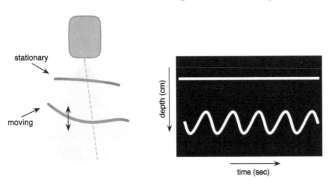

Figure 3.15 (Left) The beam is directed along the line of sight indicated by the broken line. (Right) The resulting M-mode display shows the depth of the tissue structures along this line of sight as a function of time over a period of several seconds.

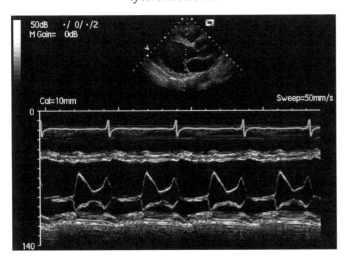

Figure 3.16. An M-mode trace showing the movement of the mitral valve leaflets.

The other one-dimensional imaging mode is the A-mode (Amplitude mode) display. Again the beam is kept in a fixed position and the machine transmits and receives along this line of sight.

However, the display simply shows echo amplitude as a function of depth, as shown in Figure 3.17.

This type of display was widely used in the early days of diagnostic ultrasound. It is rarely used now, except occasionally in some eye scans. Its attractions are its simplicity and the ability to measure the depth of the various echoes accurately.

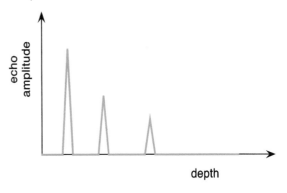

Figure 3.17 An A-mode display.

Suggested activities

1. Get an example of an image from each of the three types of probes described above (i.e. linear, curved and phased arrays). Consider where the lines of sight are in each case (i.e. where the machine directed the beam as it built up the image).

2. Examine the three images carefully for any visual clues to support your assertion regarding the lines of sight (e.g. the overall shape of the image and the position and direction of artifacts such as shadowing and enhancement, which are discussed in detail in chapter 6).

Chapter 4

Transducers

Transducer principles

The active component in an ultrasound machine's probe is the ultrasound "transducer". The term transducer means a device capable of converting energy from one form to another. For example, a microphone is a transducer since it converts sound to electrical signals.

Notice that ultrasound transducers must be bidirectional; they convert electrical pulses into transmitted ultrasound and then convert ultrasound echoes back into electrical signals.

While some naturally occurring materials (e.g. quartz) can do this, they have poor efficiency – much of the energy is lost in the conversion process. The only way to overcome this would be to expose patients to very high transmitted ultrasound power levels to compensate for the losses. Thus the development of diagnostic ultrasound had to wait until efficient ceramic transducer materials became available.

Until recently all ultrasound transducers were made from these ceramics, the most widely used being lead-zirconate-titanate. However, we will see that ceramic transducers have limited bandwidth. This is a problem, as explained in chapter 3, since a large transducer bandwidth is essential to achieving images with high resolution.

The limited bandwidth of ceramic transducers spurred the development of a new generation of materials (composites of ceramics and polymers) which can achieve much greater bandwidth. Probes made using these materials are often called "broadband" probes.

For simplicity, this section will deal only with ceramic transducers; composite transducers are quite similar in their construction and operation.

Ultrasound transducer materials are "piezoelectric".

This means that when an electrical voltage is applied to the transducer it creates a force and causes the transducer to change in size.

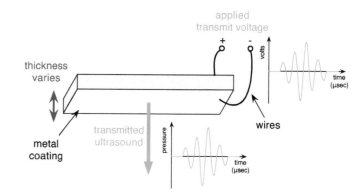

Figure 4.1 A transducer consists of a thin strip of ceramic material (grey). The front and back surfaces are coated with a very thin metallic coating (white) to which wires are attached. When an oscillating voltage is applied to the wires, the transducer oscillates in thickness, creating an ultrasound wave that travels into the patient's tissues.

Figure 4.1 shows this effect being used to transmit an ultrasound pulse. Conversely, when an ultrasound echo reaches the transducer (see Figure 4.2), the pressure variations in the echo cause the thickness of the transducer to oscillate and this produces an electrical voltage between the two wires.

This is the echo signal that the machine processes to form the ultrasound image.

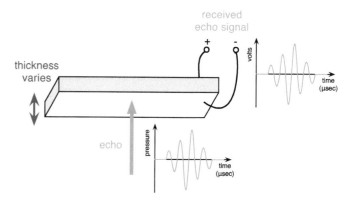

Figure 4.2 A returning echo causes the thickness of the transducer to oscillate, and this creates an electrical echo signal. Note that in reality the echo amplitude is very much smaller than the transmit pulse amplitude.

To achieve good sensitivity, ceramic transducers make use of the phenomenon of "resonance". Every transducer has a preferred frequency (known as its "resonant frequency" or sometimes its "natural frequency"). Operating the transducer at its resonant frequency ensures that its efficiency (both when transmitting and when receiving) is maximised.

As an analogy, think of an individual string in a guitar or violin. When the string is plucked or bowed it vibrates at a specific frequency and produces sound at that frequency. This is the resonant frequency of the string, and it is determined by factors such as its length, weight and tension.

What determines the resonant frequency of an ultrasound transducer? It is simply the frequency for which the thickness of the ceramic is exactly equal to half the ultrasound wavelength.

To make a transducer for a specific frequency of operation, therefore, the manufacturer must calculate the wavelength of the ultrasound at that frequency (note this is the wavelength *in the ceramic material*) and then grind the ceramic until its thickness is exactly equal to half the wavelength.

Apart from maximising the transducer's efficiency, are there other consequences of operating it at its resonant frequency?

Consider another analogy – a church bell. When the bell is hit by a hard object, it rings at its resonant frequency. An important point is that it *continues* to ring long after it was hit, gradually diminishing in loudness.

This is a characteristic of resonance.

We can therefore expect that when a transducer is used to transmit it will continue to oscillate at its resonant frequency for some time after the electrical transmit pulse has stopped. This is undesirable, since it means the duration of the transmit pulse will be extended and so the image resolution will be poor.

What can be done about this? You may notice that musicians frequently put their hands on their instrument (whether it be a drum, cymbals or a guitar string, for example) when they want it to stop sounding. This works because the hands quickly absorb energy from the instrument and bring its vibration to a stop. Pianos have felt "dampers" that touch the strings and do the same thing. Indeed the process of stopping resonant oscillations by absorbing energy is called "damping".

Ultrasound transducers are damped by placing a layer of suitable material immediately behind them (referred to as the "damping" or "backing" layer, see Figure 4.3).

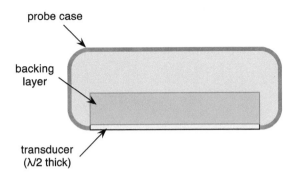

Figure 4.3 Cross-section through a typical probe, showing the transducer and backing layer.

This material (generally a plastic with additives such as metal particles) is designed so that it quickly absorbs energy and therefore keeps the transmit pulse relatively short. As an added benefit, it absorbs ultrasound energy that might otherwise travel into the probe and reflect from structures within it, causing echoes that the machine would display as if they came from the patient.

Unfortunately damping also has a negative side.

Consider a bell again. If you place your hand lightly on one side of the bell it will have a small effect on how long it rings after it is struck. If you place the hand more firmly on it, or use two hands, it will ring for a shorter time but it will also be less loud. Not surprisingly, as transducer damping is increased the same thing happens, the vibration of the transducer diminishes both in intensity and in duration. The backing layer of a transducer is therefore a compromise designed to give the *shortest pulse possible consistent with maintaining reasonable efficiency*.

Since damping a transducer makes the pulse duration shorter it follows that it must increase the transducer's bandwidth. Nevertheless, even with damping the bandwidth of a ceramic transducer is still relatively limited. In chapter 3 we saw that there is an inverse relationship between pulse duration and pulse bandwidth, and so a limited transducer bandwidth automatically lengthens the transmit pulse.

Ceramic transducers have a further serious limitation. The acoustic impedance of the transducer material is very different to the impedance of soft tissue. As discussed in the Reflection and Scattering section, this means that a large fraction of the energy striking the boundary between the transducer and the patient's tissues will be reflected, and only a small fraction will be transmitted through the boundary (see Figure 4.4). This is true both on transmission and on reception, which means that a ceramic transducer will still have an unacceptably low efficiency unless this problem can be solved.

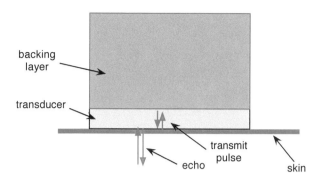

Figure 4.4 Magnified view of the interface between the transducer and the patient. Due to the large impedance mismatch between the hard ceramic transducer and the soft tissue, only a small fraction of the transmitted energy gets into the tissue, with the rest of the energy being reflected and remaining within the transducer. Similarly, most of the echo energy will be reflected back into the tissues, with only a small fraction crossing the boundary into the transducer to be converted into an echo signal.

Fortunately a technology is available to fix this, known as "impedance matching". A thin layer of material (generally a plastic) is placed directly on the front face of the transducer so that it lies between the tissues and the transducer.

The thickness of this "matching layer" must be a quarter of a wavelength and its acoustic impedance (Z_{ml}) must be:

$$Z_{ml} = \sqrt{Z_c \times Z_t}$$

where Z_c is the acoustic impedance of the ceramic transducer and Z_t is the acoustic impedance of soft tissue. The matching layer is sometimes referred to as a "quarter-wave matching layer".

The matching layer greatly improves the efficiency of energy transfer between the transducer and the tissues. As a bonus, this further dampens the transducer and so it contributes to broadening the transducer bandwidth and shortening the pulse duration.

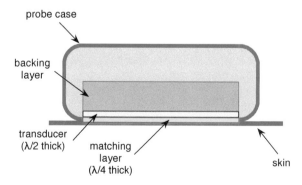

Figure 4.5 Diagram showing the transducer with its backing and matching layers.

There is one final problem that must be addressed to ensure that ultrasound can travel freely from the probe into the tissues and back to the probe. If there is even a minute amount of air between the probe and patient this will act as a very efficient reflector and little or no energy will get into the patient. Fortunately this is easily fixed using coupling gel. The gel, which is placed on the skin, forms a thin layer between the probe and skin. Its sole purpose is to eliminate all air from this region.

In the following sections we will see how array transducers are constructed and how they are used to focus and scan the ultrasound beam to create images.

Suggested activities

1. Try scanning without gel – you will find it difficult to get normal image quality.

2. Try using water as a coupling agent in place of gel. You should find that it works equally well except that it is difficult to keep it in place.

Focussing

In chapter 3 we saw that a dot is placed in the image for each echo. Its position in the image is determined by:

a) the echo arrival time – the machine uses this to calculate the depth of the point, and

b) the position of the beam.

Importantly, a reflector or scatterer will produce an echo *whenever it is within the ultrasound beam*. Since the machine cannot know whether the structure causing the echo is on the mid-line of the beam or to one side or the other of the beam, it assumes that the structure is on the mid-line and places the dot accordingly (see Figure 4.6).

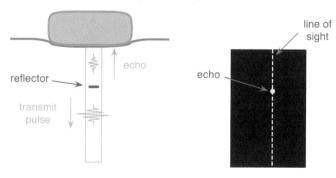

Figure 4.6 The machine places all echoes gathered by a particular beam along a line corresponding to the mid-line of the beam (generally referred to as the "line of sight").

Ideally the ultrasound beam would be very narrow (say less than 1 mm in width). In this case the echo would be positioned quite accurately. Unfortunately it is not possible to make the beam this small. If the beam is 6 mm wide, for example, a structure could be as much as 3 mm away from the mid-line and still be displayed as being on the mid-line (see Figure 4.7).

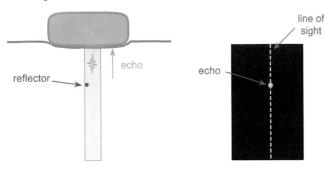

Figure 4.7 If the reflector causing the echo is on one side of the beam, its position in the image will be incorrect since it will be displayed as being on the mid-line of the beam.

Clearly we would like to get as close as possible to the ideal of having a very narrow beam. This is why focussing of the beam is an important aspect of diagnostic ultrasound.

How do we define the boundaries of the beam? Figure 4.8 shows that the edge of the beam can theoretically be defined as being the point where the intensity falls to zero. For practical reasons, a more commonly used definition of the beam boundaries is that shown in Figure 4.9, i.e. the boundaries are defined as being the points where the intensity is 20 dB below the maximum intensity. (Remember that 20 dB lower means a factor of 100 times lower than the maximum.)

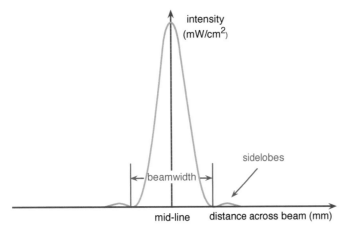

Figure 4.8 Typical intensity distribution across the beam. The intensity is maximum at the centre of the beam (i.e. on the mid-line) and becomes progressively weaker as we approach the edges of the beam. The additional "bumps" in the curve outside the beam are termed "sidelobes"; they will be discussed in a later section.

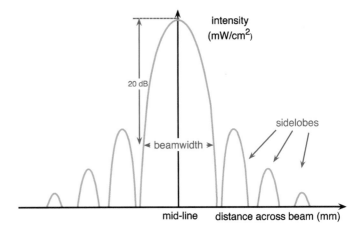

Figure 4.9 The same graph as in Figure 4.8, but using a decibel scale for the vertical axis. Notice that the sidelobes are now much more prominent than they were in Figure 4.8 due to the decibel scale.

Which machine parameters determine the beamwidth?

The most important factors are the ultrasound frequency and the size of the transducer; together they define the "diffraction limit" of the transducer, shown in Figure 4.10.

> *The diffraction limit is the narrowest possible beamwidth that can be achieved at each depth.*

It is defined by the divergence angle θ which is given by the following equation:

$$\sin\theta = \frac{1.22\lambda}{A}$$

$$\text{and so } \theta = \sin^{-1}\left(\frac{1.22\lambda}{A}\right)$$

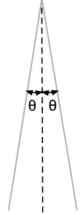

Figure 4.10 The diffraction limit of a transducer. The divergence angle θ is determined by the transducer aperture (A) and the ultrasound frequency.

Remember that the ultrasound wavelength λ is inversely proportional to frequency. We can see therefore that the divergence angle will be small – and therefore the beamwidth will be small – if the frequency is high and/or if the transducer aperture is large.

Before we look further at focussing, we need to look at unfocussed beams. Figure 4.11 shows a typical example.

In the "far zone" (or "far field") the beam is simply the diffraction limit, as described above. However, in the "near zone" (or "near field") the beam is considerably wider than the diffraction limit. Notice also that the beam narrows down to a beamwidth equal to half the transducer aperture at the point of transition from the near zone to the far zone; this is sometimes called "self-focussing".

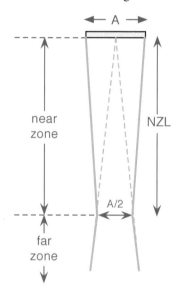

Figure 4.11 Beam pattern for an unfocussed transducer showing the near and far zones. The broken lines show the diffraction limit.

The depth at which the transition from near zone to far zone occurs is called the "near zone length" (*NZL*) or sometimes the "transition distance". The near zone length is an important parameter in the design of focussed transducers. Mathematically it is given by:

$$NZL = \frac{A^2}{4\lambda}$$

where A is the aperture and λ is the ultrasound wavelength.

> *The near zone length is important because it is only possible to focus a transducer within the near zone. To focus a transducer at a given depth, it is therefore essential that its near zone length is greater than this depth.*

The equation above shows that the near zone length will be large if the frequency is high and/or if the transducer aperture is large – the same conditions that keep the beamwidth relatively small in the far zone.

> *Focussing the beam will be most successful if the frequency is high and/or the aperture is large.*

As an example, suppose we are designing a 3 MHz transducer to focus at a depth of 20 cm. The above equation allows us to calculate that the aperture must be greater than 2 cm, since this is the smallest aperture that gives a near zone length greater than 20 cm.

There are a number of ways that a transducer can be focussed. To name two, the surface of the transducer can be curved or an acoustic lens can be placed in front of it. Both of these methods were widely used in the past before the introduction of electronic focussing. Indeed, most array transducers in use today still use a lens (as shown in Figure 4.12) to control the dimension of the ultrasound beam that is referred to as "slice thickness" (or "section thickness" or the "elevation plane").

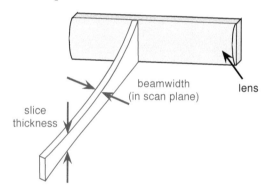

Figure 4.12 Many transducers have a cylindrical lens running the full length of the transducer. Its purpose is to focus the beam in the "slice thickness" direction, as shown here. (The beamwidth in the scan plane is not realistic in this diagram, although it is true that it is generally smaller than slice thickness.)

How does focussing actually work? We need to understand two basic concepts to answer this question – "superposition" and Huygens' principle.

Superposition deals with what happens when two (or more) ultrasound waves arrive at a single point and combine together. As Figure 4.13 shows, the result depends on their relative "phase", i.e. their relative timing. Ultrasound waves can add together constructively, destructively or somewhere in between. The amplitude of the resulting wave varies from maximum to zero depending on the phase relationship of the waves arriving at the point.

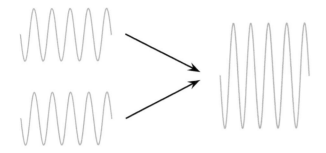

Figure 4.13 (a). Two identical waves arriving at a point "in phase" (i.e. with their peaks and troughs coinciding in time). The result is a wave with double the amplitude. This is often called "constructive interference".

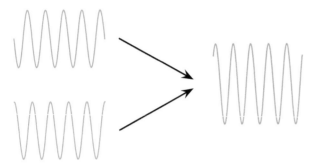

Figure 4.13 (b). Two waves with equal amplitude but different phases (in this case they are a quarter of a cycle different). The result is a wave with lower amplitude than in Figure 4.13 (a) where the two waves were in phase.

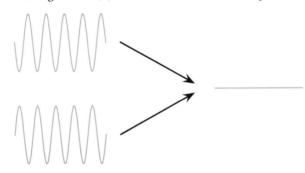

Figure 4.13 (c). Two waves with equal amplitude but opposite phase (i.e. the peaks of one coincide with the troughs of the other). The result is complete cancellation. This is often called "destructive interference".

When a transducer transmits ultrasound it is useful to consider the contribution made by each point on its face to the overall transmitted wave. Note that the energy transmitted from a *point* has no beam pattern. Instead the ultrasound spreads equally in all directions, much the same as the energy scattered by a small structure.

We can calculate the overall transmitted wave produced by the transducer by seeing how these contributions combine at each point in the tissue (see Figure 4.14). This concept is referred to as Huygens' principle.

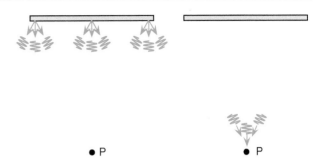

Figure 4.14 Left: For simplicity, contributions to the overall transmitted wave from just three points on the face of the transducer (the grey rectangle) are shown here. Right: The individual waves reach a point of interest in the tissue (P) at slightly different times due to the different path distances they must travel. The wave from the centre of the transducer arrives first since it is the nearest point on the transducer face to the point P.

Since the contributions from different points on the face of the transducer arrive at different times, the overall resulting transmit energy at P will be found by adding the contributions from all points on the transducer using the principle of superposition.

How can we change the transducer to get the maximum possible intensity at the point P? Figure 4.15 shows the answer – a curved transducer with P at the centre of its curvature.

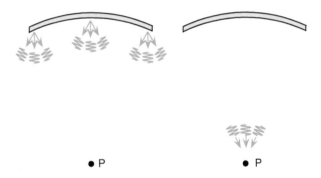

Figure 4.15 The transducer is curved, with its centre of curvature at P. This means that every point on the face of the transducer is the same distance away from P, and so all the individual waves arrive at P simultaneously.

Since the waves from all points on the face of the transducer arrive simultaneously (and therefore in phase) at the point P they will add to produce the largest possible amplitude at that point. A circle can have only one point as its centre, and P is therefore the only point where this happens. We call P the "focal point" of the transducer since it is the point where the transmitted ultrasound intensity is greatest.

What is the relationship between intensity and beamwidth? The total ultrasound power travelling along the beam is constant (ignoring attenuation).

If the beam is narrowed at a given depth, then it follows that the intensity must increase at that depth. This is so because intensity is defined as power per unit area and narrowing the beamwidth decreases the area and so increases the intensity. It also follows that the opposite statement is true – if the intensity is increased at a given depth then the beam must be narrower at that depth.

> *Thus, the focal point (or focal depth) is the depth where the intensity is greatest and the beam narrowest.*

An acoustic lens can achieve equivalent focussing to a curved transducer. The lens is made of a material (usually a plastic) with a lower propagation speed than soft tissue. Since the lens is thickest at the centre of the transducer (see Figure 4.16) it will delay the transmit signal from the centre more than from the edges of the transducer. The effect is therefore the same as if the transducer was curved.

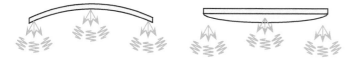

Figure 4.16 A flat transducer with a lens (right) can focus in the same way as a curved transducer (left).

Finally we have reached the point where we can look at the beam for a focussed transducer. Figure 4.17 shows an unfocussed transducer (for comparison) and then two focussed transducers of the same size and frequency as the unfocussed one.

The first thing to note is that the beam is narrowed not just at a point but over a range of depths referred to as the "focal zone". Some ultrasound machines even indicate the transmit focal zone on their display. Note also that the focal zone is longer (i.e. it covers a greater range of depths) for the transducer on the left. Secondly, notice that the beamwidth at focus is smaller for the transducer on the right, which is focussed more superficially. Thirdly, notice that at depths beyond the focal zone the beam diverges more rapidly than that for an unfocussed transducer, with this effect being worse for the transducer on the right.

The example on the right would be termed a "strongly focussed" transducer, and the one on the left a "medium focussed" transducer.

In summary, a strongly focussed transducer has a narrow beam at focus but it has only a short focal zone and the beam diverges rapidly beyond focus. Because of these limitations, it is usual for ultrasound transducers to use medium focussing.

The beamwidth at focus (bw_f) is determined by the diffraction limit:

$$bw_f = \frac{2.44 \times \lambda \times F}{A}$$

where F is the depth of focus, A is the transducer aperture and λ is the ultrasound wavelength. This reinforces the statements above:

> *The narrowest beam at focus is achieved by using the highest possible frequency and largest possible aperture.*

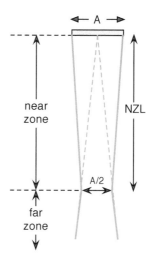

Figure 4.17 (a) Beam pattern of an unfocussed transducer. As before, the broken line is the diffraction limit of the transducer.

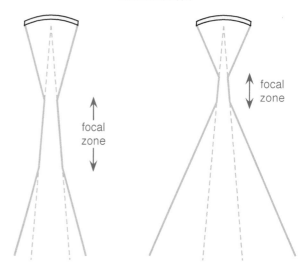

Figure 4.17 (b). Two transducers of the same size and frequency as the unfocussed transducer in Figure 4.17(a). The transducer on the right is focussed more superficially.

There are two important limitations to the discussion above. First, we have assumed continuous wave ultrasound since we have talked about a single ultrasound frequency.

What happens when a pulse is transmitted and hence a range of frequencies? The answer is that this has a relatively modest effect on everything that has been said above. It is therefore reasonable to calculate the various parameters here using the centre frequency of the pulse.

The other limitation is that we have talked only about the transmitted ultrasound beam. What about when the transducer is receiving? The answer is that the beam shape and the intensity distribution within the beam are identical, regardless of whether the transducer is transmitting or receiving.

What differs between the transmit beam and the receive beam is simply its interpretation:

1. The transmit beam defines where the transmitted energy goes and how it is distributed within the beam in terms of its intensity.

2. The receive beam defines the region of tissue from which the transducer can receive echoes (i.e. it defines where the transducer is "looking" for echoes). The intensity distribution within the beam defines how effectively the echoes are received. Echoes from the regions where the beam intensity is high (e.g. on axis around focus) will be efficiently received. Where the beam intensity is low (e.g. at the edge of the beam) the echoes will be poorly received.

In the next section, we will see how the principles in this section are applied in a modern ultrasound machine using electronic focussing.

Suggested activities

1. Look at two clinical probes and see if you can identify the lens used for controlling slice thickness.

2. Choose a clinical probe and calculate the minimum aperture it would need to have to be able to focus at a depth close to the limits of its penetration. Compare this to the overall length of the probe. What does this tell you?

3. Calculate what the beamwidth at focus would be for a 5 MHz transducer with an aperture of 2 cm focussed at a depth of 8 cm.

Array transducers

Ultrasound machines use "array" transducers. What does this term mean?

It refers to the fact that a large number of fine parallel cuts are made in the transducer material, as shown in Figure 4.18 (b). The transducer is transformed into an "array" of identical tiny transducer "elements". This array structure makes it possible to focus and steer the ultrasound beam electronically, providing much greater flexibility than other methods for achieving these functions.

The elements in an array transducer are very narrow. For the linear array shown in Figure 4.18, for example, the spacing (i.e. the distance from one element to the next) will be approximately 0.3 mm if there are a total of 256 elements.

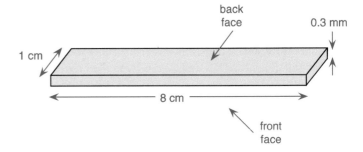

Figure 4.18 (a) A typical linear array transducer before cutting. It consists of a thin piece of ceramic material (e.g. PZT = lead-zirconate-titanate). The dimensions shown are typical for a 5 MHz transducer.

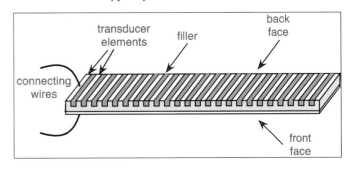

Figure 4.18 (b) The transducer is cut half-way through its thickness many times, creating a large number of narrow strips known as transducer "elements". The gaps between them are filled with an insulating material. Both the front surface of the transducer and the rear of each element are coated with a thin layer of metal (white). Each element has a separate wire connection (just one is shown) and a single wire makes contact to the whole of the front face.

Even though the cuts are just half-way through the material, they ensure that each element can operate as a separate transducer, transmitting and receiving ultrasound independent of its neighbouring elements.

As discussed in chapter 3, two other kinds of array transducer are also commonly used – curved arrays and phased arrays. Their construction is very similar to the linear array shown here.

A curved array is identical to a linear array apart from the curvature of its front face. A phased array is shorter and generally approximately square in shape (i.e. the width and length are approximately equal). A typical size would be 2 × 2 cm, with a total of either 64 or 128 elements.

These are all one dimensional probes, since the transducer is divided into a large number of elements along its length but not across its width. Both 1½D and 2D array probes are also available; in these the transducer is also divided into a number of elements across its width, as we will see later. 2D arrays are often referred to as "matrix" arrays.

Phased array transmit focussing

First we will consider transmit focussing of a phased array transducer, since this is the simplest case. All the transducer elements contribute to creating the transmit pulse, but they transmit at slightly different times, as shown in Figure 4.19.

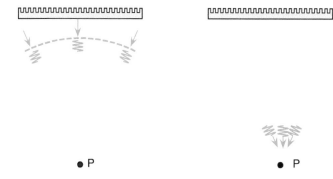

Figure 4.19 (Left) to create a beam that will focus at the point P, the outermost elements transmit first, followed by the elements adjacent to them and so on. The central element transmits last. For simplicity, only pulses transmitted by the outermost and central elements are shown. The timing of the transmit pulses is arranged so that they will lie on a circle (broken line) centred at P. (Right) as a result, the pulses arrive simultaneously and in phase at P.

Compare this with Figure 4.15. We can see that the machine has electronically simulated a curved focussed transducer. The beam will therefore be essentially identical to the beam that a curved transducer would produce. The electronics used to achieve this are shown in Figure 4.20.

If there are 128 elements in the phased array, then a total of 128 electronic delay circuits will be required. The term "channel" is used to describe the electronics associated with each element. The number of channels in a machine can range from 64 to 256 depending on the sophistication (and cost) of the machine. The user sets the depth of focus (see Figure 4.21) and the machine then calculates the necessary delays.

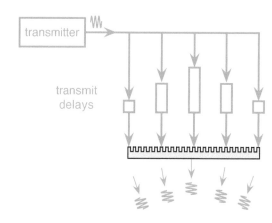

Figure 4.20 The electrical pulse from the transmitter is delivered to each transducer element via an electronic delay. The outermost elements have the shortest delays and so they transmit first. The central element has the longest delay and therefore it transmits last. Just five "channels" of the electronics are shown in this diagram. In reality there would be the same number as the number of elements in the phased array (e.g. 128).

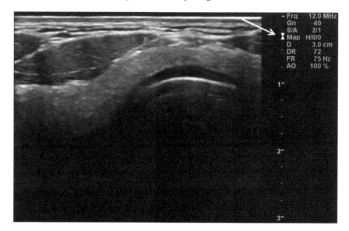

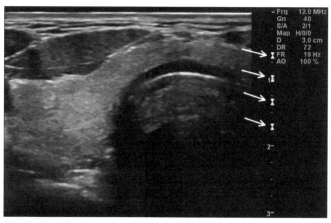

Figure 4.21 (Top) In this linear array thyroid image the depth of focus (arrow) is very shallow. Image resolution is good in the superficial tissues but the penetration is poor. The frame rate is 75 Hz. (Bottom) Multiple focus gives a more uniform image, focussed throughout its depth. Here four foci have been used (arrows). Consequently the frame rate has been reduced by a factor of four to 19 Hz.

How is the beam scanned to create a complete image? As we saw in chapter 3, a phased array probe scans the beam by steering it sequentially in a number of different directions. This is achieved using delays in a way very similar to focussing. Figure 4.22 shows a phased array producing an unfocussed beam steered to the left, and Figure 4.23 shows how steering and focussing are combined.

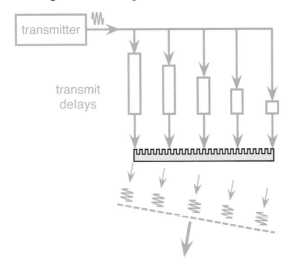

Figure 4.22 A phased array steers the beam using delays which vary in equal increments from one end of the transducer to the other. This electronically simulates tilting of the transducer, as shown by the broken line, and so the beam will be directed as shown by the arrow.

A typical phased array sweeps the beam from left to right through approximately 90°, with each line of sight (beam direction) rotated by approximately 1° relative to the previous one. Thus it will require approximately 90 transmit pulses to acquire the information for a single image.

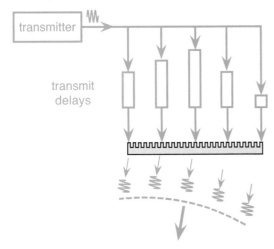

Figure 4.23 The delays required to steer the beam are added to the delays required to focus the beam. The result is a curved wavefront tilted at an angle to the transducer face (as shown by the broken line). The beam will be directed as shown by the arrow and focussed.

Phased array receive focussing

How do array transducers receive echoes?

The principle is remarkably similar to that used for transmitting. Again, electronic delays are used, in this case to delay the echo received by each element by an appropriate amount.

Consider an echo returning to a phased array transducer from a point P in the tissues. As Figure 4.24 shows, the echoes will arrive at slightly different times at each of the elements.

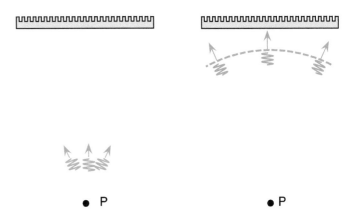

Figure 4.24 Echoes returning from the point P will arrive first at the centre element of the array and last at the outermost elements.

The block diagram in Figure 4.25 shows how the machine uses electronic delays to compensate for these different arrival times so that the echoes will be simultaneous and in phase when they are added together electronically for processing.

This ensures that the echo strength is maximised and so the receive beamwidth is minimised.

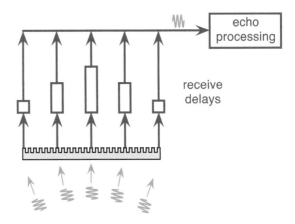

Figure 4.25 Phased array receive focussing. The echo arrives at the centre element first, so it will require the longest delay. Conversely, the echo arrives at the outermost elements last and so they will require the shortest delay.

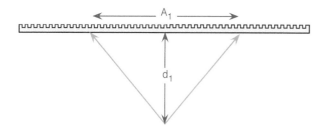

Figure 4.26 (a) When the echoes are coming from a relatively superficial depth (d₁), only the elements in the central part of the aperture are used to receive them and so the effective aperture (A₁) is relatively small.

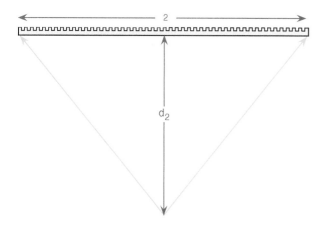

Figure 4.26 (b) As the signal comes from greater depths the number of elements used to receive the echoes increases until the full aperture (A₂) is in use.

There is one important difference between transmit focussing and receive focussing.

Whereas the transmitted beam has a single depth of focus (set by the user and displayed on the screen), receive focussing is done automatically without user intervention and it is "dynamic". This refers to the fact that at each instant the machine knows what depth the echoes are coming from (e.g. 130 μsec after the transmit pulse the echo will be coming from a depth of 10 cm).

It therefore dynamically adjusts the receive focussing delays so that at each instant the beam is correctly focussed at the depth from which the echoes are coming. This is known as "dynamic focussing".

Further, the number of elements used to receive the echoes (and hence the receive aperture) is dynamically varied with depth as shown in Figure 4.26. This is known as "dynamic aperture".

Linear array

Next we will look at how a linear array differs from the phased array.

As Figure 4.27 shows, a typical linear array contains 256 (or more) elements.

Each beam is created using a subset of these elements (generally a group of 128 elements).

The beam is scanned by stepping it along the face of the transducer. The last line of sight uses elements 129 to 256 and thus the image will contain a total of 129 lines of sight.

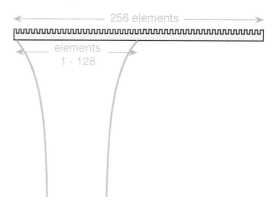

Figure 4.27 (a) A linear array transducer with 256 elements. Each beam is created using 128 elements. The first line of sight (beam position) uses elements 1 to 128.

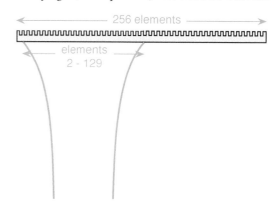

Figure 4.27 (b) The second line of sight uses elements 2 to 129, and so it is displaced to the right relative to the first beam by an amount equal to the element spacing (a fraction of a millimetre).

Since there is no steering of the beam in the "standard" grey scale imaging mode of operation for the linear array, all the beams are parallel and at 90° to the transducer face, as shown in Figure 4.28 (a).

However, there are other modes of operation which do require the beam to be steered, as shown in Figures 4.28 (b), (c) and (d).

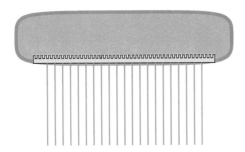

Figure 4.28 (a) Scan pattern for a linear array operating in its standard imaging mode.

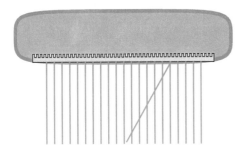

Figure 4.28 (b) In pulsed Doppler mode the direction of the imaging beams is unchanged but the Doppler beam may be steered to ensure that the angle between the beam and the vessel is appropriate, as discussed later.

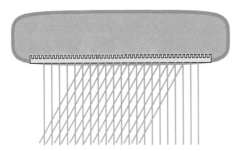

Figure 4.28 (c) In colour Doppler mode all of the colour lines may be steered to achieve an appropriate Doppler angle, as shown here. As with pulsed Doppler mode, the direction of the imaging lines is unchanged.

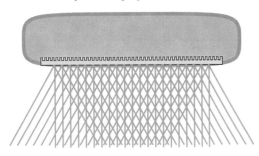

Figure 4.28 (d) In spatial compound scanning several grey scale images are created, each with a different beam steering direction. The images are then combined to produce a single composite image. As discussed in chapter 12, the benefits of this mode of operation include more complete imaging of tissue boundaries and smoothing of the speckle in soft tissue areas.

Curved array

A curved array is identical in operation to a linear array except that the curvature causes the beams to change direction as they step along the transducer face, and hence there is a radial component to its scan pattern.

1½D and 2D arrays

As mentioned earlier, standard linear, curved and phased array transducers are one dimensional (1D), since they are divided into a large number of elements along their length.

In recent years both 1½D and 2D transducers have come into use. These are divided into elements across the width of the transducer as well, as shown in Figure 4.29.

The small number of elements across the width of 1½D array transducers means that they are limited in their capabilities when compared with full 2D ("matrix") arrays. Nevertheless, 1½D arrays can improve the ultrasound beam's "slice thickness" (see the next section) using the dynamic aperture technique described above.

True 2D array transducers have two major advantages.

First, they can focus the beam in the slice thickness direction using both dynamic aperture and conventional beamforming with delays.

Secondly, they can be used to steer the entire scan plane in a number of different directions, thus sweeping it through a volume of tissue. 2D arrays can thus be used for 3D imaging, eliminating the need for manual or mechanical scanning. Also, since electronic scanning and focussing can be extremely fast, 2D arrays have made it possible for the first time to produce 3D images in real time.

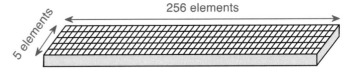

Figure 4.29 (a) A 1½D array transducer has a small number of cuts dividing it into elements across its width.

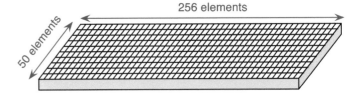

Figure 4.29 (b) A 2D (or "matrix") transducer has a larger number of elements across the width and therefore a very large number of elements in total.

Naturally a price is paid for these improvements. 2D probes are more bulky and expensive than conventional probes.

Suggested activities

1. Consider the 5 MHz linear array in Figure 4.18 and assume it consists of 256 elements of which 128 are used to form each individual beam (as shown in Figure 4.27). If the beam is focussed at a depth of 5 cm, calculate the beamwidth at focus.

2. Assuming the width of the transducer is 1 cm as shown in Figure 4.18, calculate the slice thickness at a depth of 5 cm (assuming the lens controlling slice thickness is focussed at this depth).

3. Assuming that the maximum depth of penetration for the above transducer is 10 cm and that there are 128 lines of sight in each image, calculate the minimum time needed to produce one image and hence calculate the maximum number of images each second (i.e. the frame rate).

Beams, image quality and artifacts

In the last two sections of this chapter you have been introduced to the nature of the ultrasound beam and the electronic methods used to focus and scan it through tissues. In this section we will explore the limitations of beamforming and some of the artifacts (misleading appearances) related to these limitations. In particular we will look at beamwidth, slice thickness, sidelobes and grating lobes.

Beamwidth

Figure 4.30 shows how the ultrasound machine displays an object as though it were on the centre-line of the beam (the line of sight), no matter where in the beam it actually lies.

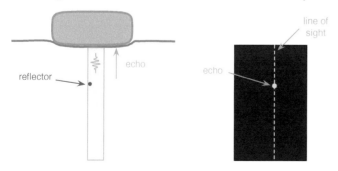

Figure 4.30 If a reflector causing an echo is on one side of the beam, its position in the image will be incorrect since it will be displayed as being on the mid-line of the beam.

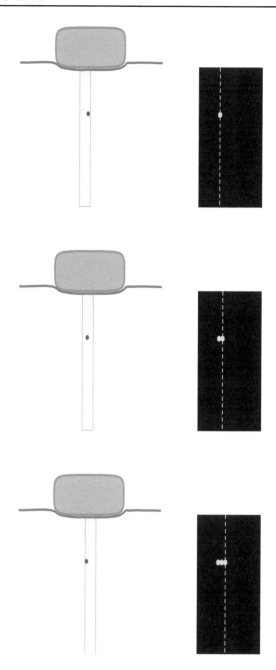

Figure 4.31 A time sequence showing three successive beam positions as the probe scans the tissues from left to right. The object produces an echo each time, and so it is displayed. The displayed position is slightly different each time and so it is smeared out laterally. In reality the lines of sight are more closely spaced than shown here and so the dots in the image merge to form a line.

Figure 4.31 shows an important consequence of this. As the beam is scanned it steps from one end of the probe to the other. Since the distance that the beam moves each time is very small, a number of different beam positions (lines of sight) will "see" the object, and hence it will be displayed several times in the image in different positions. While the depth remains constant, the lateral position will change each time.

> *Thus a single object will be "smeared out" laterally by an amount equal to the beamwidth.*

Generally the beamwidth is significant in size (several millimetres), and so there will be substantial degradation of the image. (For a 4 MHz transducer with a 2 cm aperture focussed at a depth of 8 cm, for example, the beamwidth at focus will be approximately 4 mm; at other depths it will be larger than this.) An example is shown in Figure 4.32.

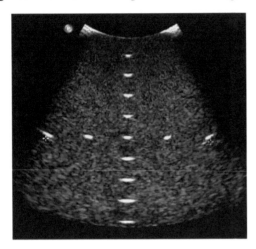

Figure 4.32 (a) Image of an ultrasound phantom showing point reflectors displayed as bright lines. The lines are smeared laterally due to the beamwidth.

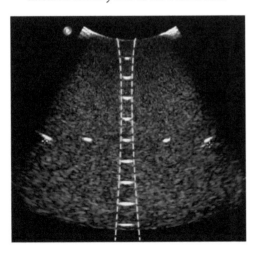

Figure 4.32(b) The beam pattern of the transducer has been superimposed on the image.

This is a scan of a tissue equivalent phantom containing a number of equally spaced point targets (pieces of fine nylon fishing line scanned in cross section). The lateral smearing of the bright reflections due to the beamwidth is clearly seen. Notice that the smearing is perpendicular to the beam direction and hence these lines are not horizontal except in the centre of the image. It is possible to determine the general shape of the beam from this image, as shown.

A clinical image showing beamwidth effects is shown in Figure 4.33.

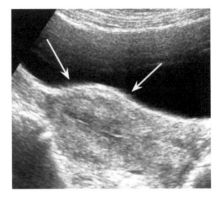

Figure 4.33 This image shows the "whiskery" appearance typically seen where boundaries between tissue and fluid are scanned at angles other than perpendicular incidence. Every point on the boundary has been smeared laterally, just like the point objects in Figure 4.32, because of the finite width of the beam.

The images in Figures 4.32 and 4.33 highlight the way beamwidth effects make it difficult to locate precisely where a specific point object (Figure 4.32) or boundary (Figure 4.33) is located. This will obviously reduce the clarity of the image and degrade the accuracy of measurements.

> *In short, beamwidth degrades image resolution, and the larger the beamwidth the worse this effect will be.*

Slice thickness

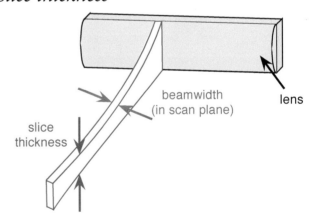

Figure 4.34 A lens focusses the beam in the slice thickness direction. (The beamwidth within the scan plane is not realistic in this diagram, although it is true that it is generally smaller than slice thickness.)

Earlier you were introduced to the concept of the "slice thickness" dimension of the ultrasound beam (sometimes called "section thickness" or the "elevation plane"), as shown in Figure 4.34.

Ideally we would like the slice thickness to be very narrow, in which case our image would represent a thin slice through the patient's anatomy, as shown in Figure 4.35.

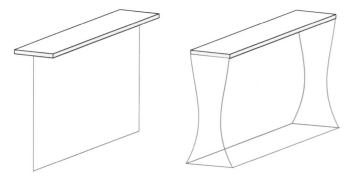

Figure 4.35 (Left) The scan plane would be like a thin slice through the patient's tissues in the ideal case where the slice thickness is very small. (Right) In reality the slice thickness is substantial, and so the image contains contributions from throughout the volume swept by the beam. This will cause slice thickness or "partial volume" artifacts, which will be discussed later.

Sidelobes

The concept of sidelobes was also introduced earlier in this chapter. It refers to additional beams that occur either side of the desired ultrasound beam (see Figure 4.36).

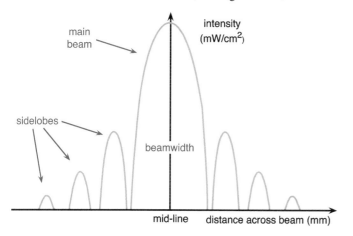

Figure 4.36 The intensity distribution across the beam at a given depth. (The use of a decibel scale for the vertical axis makes the sidelobes appear more prominent than if a linear scale had been used.)

Although they are generally weaker than the main beam by 20 dB (a factor of 100) or more, they are still capable of contributing echoes to the image and can therefore cause artifacts.

Figure 4.37 shows a curved array transducer with its main beam pointing straight down and a set of three sidelobes on either side.

Since the machine cannot know that the echo from the object comes from a sidelobe, it displays it along the midline of the main beam.

As the beam is scanned, the object will therefore be imaged in its correct location by the main beam and also to the left and right of its true location by the sidelobes. This is referred to as a sidelobe artifact.

Figure 4.38 shows a clinical example of a sidelobe artifact. Note that, since this is a curved array, the artifacts are curved (i.e. they are at a constant depth from the face of the transducer).

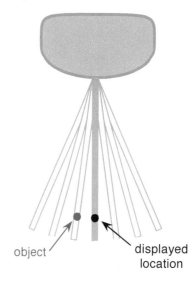

Figure 4.37 Transducer showing main beam and sidelobes. A strong reflecting object may produce a detectable echo when it falls within a sidelobe. The machine is unable to tell that the echo has come from the sidelobe, and displays it (black dot) as if it had come from the main beam.

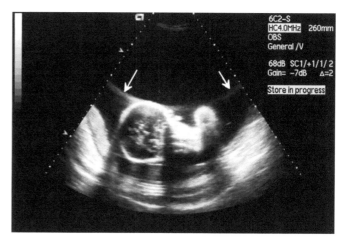

Figure 4.38 Example of a sidelobe artifact (arrows). The strongly reflective boundary between the fetus and amniotic fluid has been replicated (with reduced intensity) to the left and right of its true position.

Fortunately there is a technological solution, "apodisation", which greatly reduces the problem. On both transmission of the pulse and reception of the echoes, the machine de-emphasises the contribution of the outer transducer elements in the aperture. Thus the transmit pulse amplitude is reduced for these elements (compared with the amplitude used for the other elements) and the receive amplification applied to signals coming from these outer elements is also lower than for the rest. This significantly reduces the amplitude of the sidelobes and so makes sidelobe artifacts less noticeable. The penalty is a slight increase in the beamwidth of the main beam.

Grating lobes

A grating lobe is simply another type of sidelobe. However, grating lobes are particularly important because, *if they occur*, they are higher in amplitude than the normal sidelobes described above. As with normal sidelobes there is a technological fix for this type of sidelobe. Better yet, it *eliminates* grating lobes, whereas apodisation only *reduces* normal sidelobes.

So, what is a grating lobe and how can it occur? Figures 4.39 and 4.40 give the answer to these questions. Figure 4.39 shows a transducer with the main beam directed vertically into the tissues and a grating lobe directed at a specific angle either side of this beam.

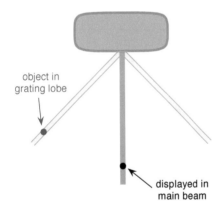

Figure 4.39 If a grating lobe exists it will have comparable strength to the main beam. Objects in the grating lobe will be displayed as if they are in the main beam.

Examining the situation closely (see Figure 4.40) we find that geometry is the key to how the grating lobe occurs.

If the pulses travelling in a particular direction from two adjacent transducer elements are exactly one cycle apart they will add together constructively, creating a grating lobe. (Recall the discussion of superposition earlier in this chapter.) Notice that the amplitude of the grating lobe pulse is not much less than the amplitude of the pulse in the main beam.

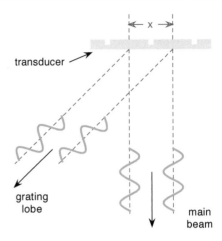

Figure 4.40 (a) The geometry required for a grating lobe to be created. Transmit pulses sent along the main beam from adjacent transducer elements will arrive simultaneously. Pulses along the grating lobe will arrive exactly one cycle apart.

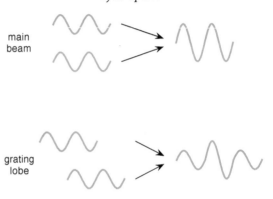

Figure 4.40 (b) In this diagram both sets of pulses are in phase and so they will combine constructively, forming the main beam and grating lobe.

What is the technical fix for this problem? It is simply to ensure that the geometry of the transducer does not allow the situation shown here. We will not present the details, but simply state that grating lobes cannot occur so long as the distance from one transducer element to the next (x in Figure 4.40 (a)) is less than half the wavelength. Most transducers are designed so that this rule is obeyed.

Suggested activities

Looking carefully at some clinical images:

1. Try to identify the "whiskery" effect caused by the beamwidth, particularly where boundaries between tissue and fluid have been scanned at an oblique angle (i.e. non-perpendicular incidence).

2. See if you can find any examples of sidelobe artifacts. Again, these will most easily be seen in echo-free areas (e.g. the gallbladder and urinary bladder).

Chapter 5

Ultrasound instrumentation

Introductory comments

In this chapter we will look at how the ultrasound machine works – how it creates transmitted ultrasound pulses and converts the received echoes into images. This will also allow us to discuss the controls available to the user and their purpose.

A few general comments may be useful first.

Ultrasound machines vary substantially in how they achieve the various functions they perform. This is highlighted by the variety of equipment available today, ranging from large full-featured machines to tiny pocket-sized ones.

Over recent years we have seen a steady increase in the use of digital processing, and this will continue. Most ultrasound machines now digitise the ultrasound signal early in the sequence of processing steps and the remainder of the processing is then done digitally (i.e. using computer chips and under the control of software).

This has the great advantage that software is easily changed, and so machines can be upgraded simply by upgrading their software. New functions can be incorporated by adding new software, and existing functions can be improved. As mentioned in chapter 1, innovation and change are constant features of the ultrasound industry.

Digital systems are also inherently stable, unlike the "analogue" (non-digital) equipment of 20 years ago whose performance changed with time, necessitating regular testing and recalibration.

Digital systems can even monitor themselves, keeping a log of any problems to help the service technicians when they do their regular system maintenance.

While much of the terminology relating to ultrasound machines has become standardised, variations can still be seen between different authors. Furthermore, equipment manufacturers often use their own terminology for a given function as a way of differentiating themselves in the market.

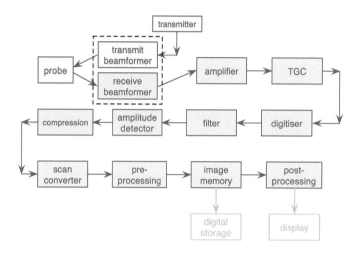

Figure 5.1 Block diagram of a typical ultrasound machine.

The block diagram in Figure 5.1 may be very daunting at first glance. However, the components in it will be addressed one by one and so (hopefully) you will be able to build up your knowledge of the machine in easy steps. For convenience we will deal here only with "standard" grey scale imaging. Specialised modes such as spatial compound scanning and harmonics will be discussed in chapter 12.

The machine's front end

In this section we will look at what is often termed the "front end" of the machine – the probe, transmitter, beamformer and amplifier (see Figure 5.2).

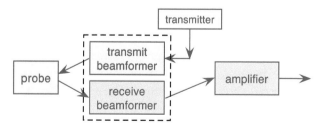

Figure 5.2 Block diagram showing the machine's "front end".

Probe

The construction of the transducer and probe has been covered already in chapter 4. A few additional comments are needed, however. A typical array transducer uses 128 transducer elements to transmit and receive at any one time. Generally this means that there will need to be at least 128 wires within the transducer cable connecting the probe to the machine.

This explains why the cable is so bulky and why there are such a large number of individual connectors in the plug connecting the probe to the machine (as shown in Figure 5.3).

Many probes contain some electronics (e.g. switching circuits to select which elements are in use at a given time), which may cause them to become warm with use.

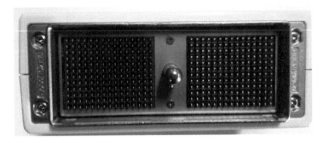

Figure 5.3 A typical probe connector plug showing the large number of connections needed between the probe and the ultrasound machine.

Transmitter

The transmitter generates the electronic transmit signal that is applied to the transducer. It is programmed by the machine's software to produce a transmit pulse of the correct frequency, pulse duration and amplitude and with an appropriate PRF. Like all the machine's settings, these are initially set at default values by the machine when the probe and examination type are selected at the start of the examination. The user has the ability to change a number of these settings subsequently, however.

Generally the amplitude of the transmit pulse can be decreased or increased using the Power control. Since increased power means increased patient exposure to ultrasound energy, the power should be increased *only* if other measures (e.g. increasing the gain and using a lower frequency) have not been sufficient to get the required information.

Often it is possible to change the frequency (within the limits of the probe's overall bandwidth) using a control that selects either penetration (relatively low frequency) or resolution (higher frequency) as a priority.

For example, a C7-3 probe would have an overall bandwidth of 3 - 7 MHz. On the "general" setting it might transmit at 5 MHz, while it may drop to 4 MHz on the "penetration" setting and increase to 6 MHz on the "resolution" setting.

As discussed in chapter 3, the machine must wait until all detectable echoes have returned to the transducer before it transmits again. The Pulse Repetition Frequency is therefore limited by the depth of penetration (which in turn depends on the frequency being used).

The machine therefore selects a PRF that is as high as possible consistent with meeting this criterion, since this will maximise the speed of image acquisition and hence the frame rate. Altering some machine settings (e.g. reducing the depth and/or zooming during scanning) can allow the machine to increase the PRF further.

Beamformer

The function and general structure of the transmit and the receive beamformers has been discussed already in chapter 4. In both cases a series of delay circuits is used – one delay for each transducer element in use at that time. Thus a typical beamformer will contain 128 transmit delays and 128 receive delays.

The transmit beamformer (see Figure 5.4) contains delays which serve to delay the transmit pulse for each element by an appropriate amount to achieve the desired depth of focus (and beam direction, if beam steering is being used). These delay values are programmed by the machine's software, based on the user's selection of the depth of focus.

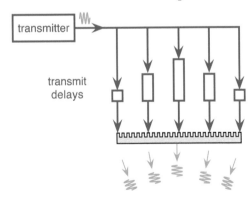

Figure 5.4 Diagram of the transmit beamformer showing just 5 transducer elements (and hence just 5 transmit delays) for simplicity. In reality 128 elements are commonly used.

The receive beamformer (see Figure 5.5) delays the received echo signal from each transducer element by an appropriate amount so that the beam is focussed at the depth from which the echo is coming.

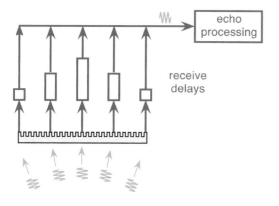

Figure 5.5 Block diagram of the receive beamformer. The delays change continuously to achieve dynamic focussing.

These delays are continuously altered by the machine's software to achieve dynamic focussing so that the focal depth tracks the depth that the echoes are coming from as they progressively come from deeper and deeper tissues. There are no user controls for the receive focussing function.

Amplifier

The echo signals are very low level, generally ranging from microvolts to millivolts in amplitude. They therefore need to be amplified to a higher level to facilitate subsequent processing and minimise the effect of electronic noise (which is present in all electronic systems). The amount of amplification (or the "gain") is preset by the machine, but the user can change it to vary the overall displayed intensity of the image using the machine's Gain control.

Suggested activities

1. Consider the machine that you use and the controls that relate to this section.

2. Alter each of these controls to see its effect on the image.

Signal processing

This section deals with the next sequence of processing steps: TGC, digitisation, filtering, amplitude detection and dynamic range compression (see Figure 5.6).

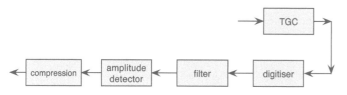

Figure 5.6 The signal processing components of the ultrasound machine.

TGC

As discussed in chapter 2, both the transmitted ultrasound pulse and the returning echoes are attenuated as they pass through tissue. For example, at a frequency of 6 MHz in normal soft tissue the intensity will be reduced by 3 dB (i.e. it will be halved) for each centimetre of travel.

Given that this applies equally to the transmit pulse and the echo, the received echo will be reduced by 6 dB (i.e. by a factor of four) for each centimetre of depth into the patient. If this was not compensated, echo information would be visible in the image for superficial tissues but it would quickly fade with depth and deeper tissues would not be seen in the image (see Figure 5.7).

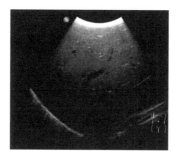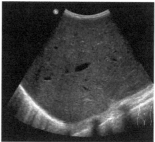

Figure 5.7 (Left) image without adequate TGC, showing loss of echoes with depth. (Right) with the TGC adjusted correctly the intensity is similar throughout the display.

The ultrasound machine therefore provides the TGC function (Time Gain Compensation, occasionally called Depth Gain Compensation). This applies a time-varying gain to the signals, beginning with a relatively low gain and increasing steadily with time as the echoes come from greater depths.

In the example mentioned above, the gain would increase at a rate of 6 dB for each 13 μsec, since this is the time that elapses for each centimetre of depth (see Figure 5.8).

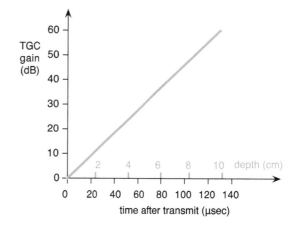

Figure 5.8 For a 6 MHz transducer, the TGC function will increase the gain by 6 dB for each centimetre of depth, that is by 6 dB for each 13 μsec of elapsed time.

This would be adequate if all tissues had the same attenuation. Unfortunately tissues are quite variable in their attenuation (compare soft tissue with liquids, for example) and so it is necessary for the user to fine-tune the TGC function to account for these variations and achieve a uniform grey scale intensity at all depths. The function is generally provided in the form of a series of slider controls, as shown in Figure 5.9.

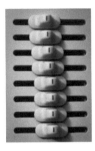

Figure 5.9 Photograph of the TGC sliders on the control panel of an ultrasound machine.

Each corresponds to a specific depth in the image. Moving a slider to the right will increase the gain at the corresponding depth, while moving it to the left will decrease the gain (see Figure 5.10). This is one of the controls that most frequently need adjusting as patients are scanned.

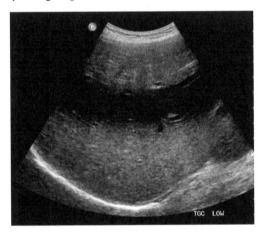

Figure 5.10 (a) Incorrect setting of the TGC control has created a dark band part-way through the liver.

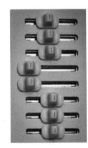

Figure 5.10 (b) Two of the TGC sliders were moved to the left, causing the misleading appearance seen in the image above.

Digitisation

Up to this point in the processing, the echo signals are time-varying voltages, commonly referred to as "analogue" signals. They are converted to "digital" signals by an analogue-to-digital converter (generally written as "A/D converter").

A digital signal is a series of binary (digital) numbers at regular time intervals. Each number represents the value of the analogue signal at the instant when it was created (see Figure 5.11). The sequence of numbers thus represents the signal, and its variation with time, in a form that is understood by the machine's software.

For example, the analogue signal may be measured by the A/D converter once every 0.1 µsec. The digitised signal will then consist of ten million binary numbers ("samples") each second. Importantly, as long as the number of samples each second (the "sampling rate") is sufficiently high, no information is lost in this digitisation process.

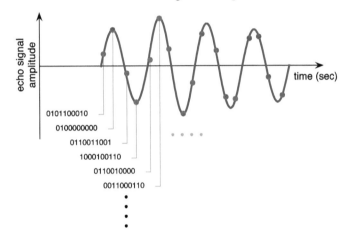

Figure 5.11 The amplitude of the echo signal is measured ("sampled") at regular intervals (indicated by the red dots) and converted into a sequence of binary numbers.

As discussed in the previous section, once the ultrasound signal has been converted to digital form it is readily processed by the machine using digital (i.e. computer) circuits and software. (Digitisation of analogue signals is common. Music signals are digitised for storage in CD or MP3 format and television signals are digitised for storage on a DVD.)

Filter

Unfortunately all electronic systems produce electronic "noise", a random signal uniformly spread across all frequencies. If this noise is allowed to appear in the image it will be seen as small echoes randomly distributed throughout the image (often termed "snow"). It is therefore important not to increase the gain to the point where noise is displayed.

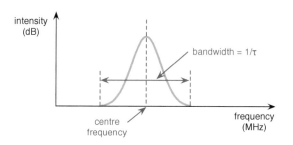

Figure 5.12 (a). The spectrum of the ultrasound signal is determined by the frequency and duration of the transmitted ultrasound pulse. The centre frequency is equal to the transmit frequency and the bandwidth is equal to the reciprocal of the pulse duration (τ).

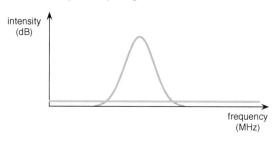

Figure 5.12 (b). Prior to filtering, the electronic noise (horizontal line) has equal intensity at all frequencies.

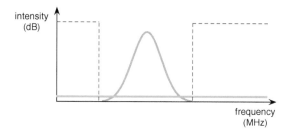

Figure 5.12 (c). The filter (broken lines) will remove all frequencies above and below the bandwidth of the ultrasound signal.

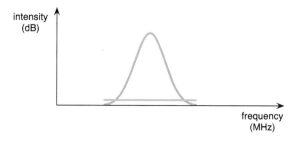

Figure 5.12 (d) After filtering, only noise at frequencies within the frequency range of the ultrasound signal is left. The total energy of the noise is reduced, and so its amplitude is reduced relative to the signal. Echoes whose amplitude is equal to that of the noise or less cannot be displayed, since increasing the gain to make these echoes visible would make the noise visible as well.

This means that echoes whose amplitude is equal to that of the noise or less cannot be displayed, since increasing the gain to make these echoes visible would make the noise visible as well. Thus processing that reduces the amplitude of the noise relative to the echo signals will improve the machine's ability to display low-level echoes and so it will improve the depth of penetration.

The filtering step in the machine's processing addresses this by removing noise at all frequencies outside the range of frequencies present in the echo signal bandwidth. Since this removes much of the noise without removing any of the echo signal, it achieves our goal of reducing the noise relative to the signal.

How does the ultrasound machine know which frequencies it can safely remove? We saw in chapter 3 that the spectrum of the ultrasound transmit pulse – and therefore also of the received echoes – is easily determined from the frequency and pulse duration of the transmit pulse as shown in Figure 5.12.

Amplitude detection

Recall that the brightness displayed at any given point in the image is determined by the strength of the echo.

This step of the processing therefore determines the amplitude of the signal and discards the more detailed information relating to the ultrasound frequency (see Figure 5.13).

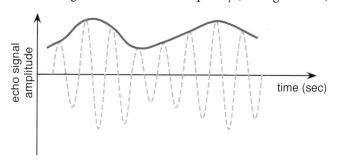

Figure 5.13 Amplitude detection. The machine calculates the amplitude of the echo (solid line) which will determine the brightness of the image at each point. The detailed ultrasound frequency information (broken line) is discarded.

Dynamic range compression

The term "dynamic range" refers to the overall range of echo intensities used to form the image.

Formally, it is defined as the ratio of the strongest to the weakest echo and it is generally measured in decibels (see the Mathematics review section.)

Thus:

$$\text{dynamic range} = 10 \times \log\left[\frac{I_{max}}{I_{min}}\right]$$

where I_{max} is the intensity of the strongest echo and I_{min} is the intensity of the weakest echo. As an example, a ratio of 1,000,000 to 1 would be a dynamic range of 60 dB.

Ultrasound echoes can range from very weak echoes caused by the scattering of ultrasound by soft tissue to very strong echoes caused by the reflection of ultrasound from tissue boundaries. The dynamic range of the echoes is therefore large – typically 60 dB or more.

As already discussed, the strength of each echo determines the brightness of the dot that represents it in the image.

A grey scale is used, with black representing a complete absence of echoes and white representing the strongest echoes. The various shades of grey represent the various echo intensities within the dynamic range.

Now that we have established that the dynamic range of the ultrasound signal is 60 dB or more, we need to ask the following question. What is the dynamic range of grey scale intensities that the eye can perceive when viewing an image?

Perhaps surprisingly, the answer to this is that human vision is limited to a dynamic range of at most 30 dB (i.e. an intensity range of 1,000 to 1) in this situation.

Thus we see that there is an inherent mismatch between the relatively limited dynamic range that can be displayed in the image and the much larger dynamic range of the ultrasound signal.

This is addressed by the "dynamic range compression" (or simply "compression") function of the machine.

A "compression curve" specifies the grey scale value to be displayed for each echo, as shown in Figure 5.14. The broken lines, for example, show that an echo 30 dB above the minimum intensity will be displayed as a near-white value just 5 dB below the maximum brightness of the display.

Note that the compression curve is not a straight line. This means that the low-level echoes from soft tissue scattering (which occupy approximately the first 30 dB of the signal dynamic range) are displayed using the majority of the grey scale range while the strong echoes from interfaces (occupying approximately the top 30 dB of the signal dynamic range) are displayed using just the top 5 dB of the grey scale range.

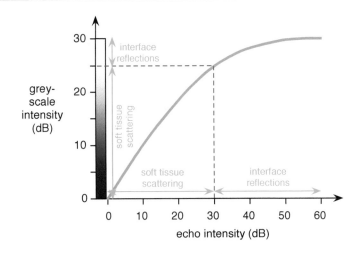

Figure 5.14 Compression curve showing how the machine translates the intensity of each echo into a grey scale intensity on the display. (Both the echo and grey scale intensity values are measured in dB relative to the lowest level.)

This is intentional. The curve is designed to allocate the majority of the grey scale levels to showing variations in the echoes from scattering, which means that all the strong echoes will be displayed as white or close to white.

Why is this? Variations in the strength of echoes from soft tissue are often very important clinically. They help the user to distinguish between different soft tissues and can also be useful to differentiate between normal and abnormal tissues in homogeneous organs such as the liver. In contrast, variations in the strength of the echoes from interfaces are often due to variations in the orientation of the interfaces relative to the beam, rather than variations in tissue properties, and hence they are of little clinical significance.

The curve shown in Figure 5.14 compresses 60 dB of signal dynamic range into 30 dB of grey scale dynamic range. In some clinical situations (e.g. echocardiography) better image quality will be obtained using a more limited range of echo intensities to form the image.

Figure 5.15 shows a compression curve which compresses just 40 dB of signal dynamic range into the 30 dB of grey scale dynamic range.

Strong echoes from interfaces (the top 30 dB of the echo range) are now allocated a larger portion of the grey scale range – approximately half – with the soft tissue echoes displayed using the lower half of the grey scale range. The lowest 20 dB of scattering echoes will not be displayed at all.

Why would you want to discard some of the low-level echoes?

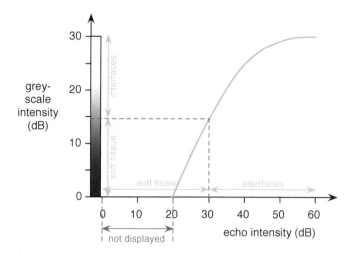

Figure 5.15 Compression curve set to display just 40 dB of echo signal dynamic range. The weakest echoes (spanning the first 20 dB of the dynamic range) are not displayed.

In echocardiography the target organ consists of relatively strong tissue echoes (from the heart walls, valves etc) and blood-filled regions which should be echo-free. Unfortunately low-level echoes occur throughout the image due to artifacts. These artifacts are visible – and therefore distracting – when they occur in the areas that should be echo-free. It is therefore common in echocardiography to use a compression curve such as that shown in Figure 5.15 to eliminate the low-level echoes and so "clean up" the image.

Ultrasound machines therefore offer a range of compression curves. As with other controls, a specific curve is preselected by the machine when probe and application area are selected at the start of each examination.

However, the user can select different curves using the machine's controls. (This control may be called "compression", "dynamic range", "contrast" or "curves".) The machine may indicate the dynamic range setting in dB (this will be the dynamic range of the signals that are being used to form the image) or as a "curve" setting (C_1, C_2 etc.). Thus the curve in Figure 5.14 provides a dynamic range of 60 dB while that in Figure 5.15 reduces the dynamic range to 40 dB.

Figure 5.16 shows the effect on an abdominal image of changing the dynamic range setting. With low dynamic range the image is more black-and-white in appearance (often described as "contrasty") and there may be areas where the echoes have dropped out completely and so information has been lost. However, artifact echoes are largely absent.

With high dynamic range, the soft tissue image texture is more uniform, but artifact echoes are now evident, particularly in the large vessels in the lower portion of the image.

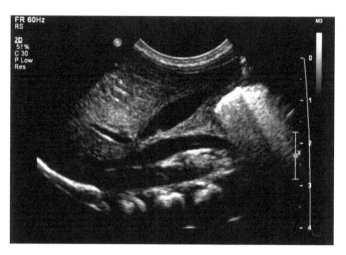

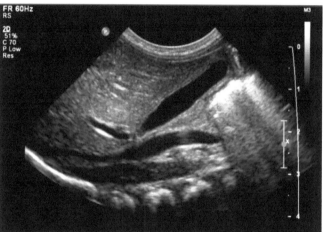

Figure 5.16 (Top) an abdominal scan acquired using a low dynamic range setting. (Bottom) the same region scanned using a higher dynamic range setting.

Suggested activities

1. Watch an experienced sonographer scanning patients. Note the use of the TGC control and its effect on the image.

2. Identify which control on your machine is used to change the dynamic range compression, and how its setting is displayed on the screen. Note whether it sets to the same default setting for different types of examination. Experiment with altering the dynamic range and carefully note the effect on the image.

Image processing

In the previous two sections you have seen how the machine acquires the echo signal and amplifies, digitises and filters it. The amplitude has then been extracted and the dynamic range compressed. The echoes are now ready to be stored and displayed as an image.

In this section we will examine the final sequence of processing steps in the machine, shown in Figure 5.17.

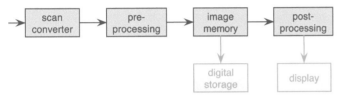

Figure 5.17 The image processing portion of the ultrasound machine.

Scan converter

The main purpose of the scan converter is to store the image in a suitable format in the image memory so that it can be displayed.

As we will see shortly, the image memory consists of a series of rows and columns of digital memory locations. It is thus rectangular in shape, reflecting the rectangular shape of the image display.

The echo information, however, is acquired one line of sight at a time. The lines of sight have widely varying orientation depending on the type of probe being used. Their position relative to the image area will be further modified by the depth and zoom settings of the machine (see Figures 5.18 and 5.19 and discussed in more detail below).

Thus the primary task of the scan converter is to place each echo in its correct location in the image memory, taking into account these factors.

Depending on the probe's scan pattern, its "line density" (i.e. the spacing of its lines of sight) and factors such as depth and zoom, the lines of sight may or may not pass through every storage location ("pixel") in the image memory.

If echo information is not written to some pixels, the image will be degraded substantially (as shown in Figure 5.20).

The scan converter therefore uses a mathematical technique known as "interpolation" to fill the gaps between the scan lines with appropriate values. The visual quality of the image is greatly improved as a result.

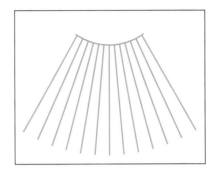

Figure 5.18 Scan pattern of a curved array probe. The scan converter must calculate the position and direction of each of the lines of sight so that individual echoes will be displayed in the correct locations.

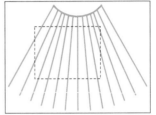 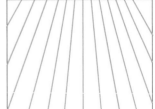

Figure 5.19 (Left) if zoom is applied while scanning then only those scan lines that fall within the zoom box (broken lines) will be acquired and stored in the image memory. (Right) zooming changes the scan pattern of the stored image dramatically.

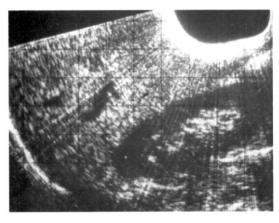

Figure 5.20 An early abdominal scan showing visual degradation of the image when individual lines of sight are visible. In modern ultrasound machines the scan converter fills the spaces between the lines of sight with appropriate values.

Pre-processing

The term "pre-processing" refers to changes made to the echo information immediately *before it is stored as an image*. Once these changes have been made and the image has been stored the changes cannot be "undone". This is in contrast to post-processing, whose effects are reversible.

Examples of pre-processing include:

- depth
- zoom
- persistence
- compound imaging
- extended field of view imaging

The depth control simply adjusts how many centimetres depth of tissue is displayed on the screen. Reducing the depth means that for each line of sight the echo data will be written to the image for a shorter time. This may allow the machine to increase the PRF, which would mean that the frame rate would also increase.

In general the user adjusts the depth control so that all of the tissues of interest are displayed in the image and so that they occupy as much of the image area as possible.

The zoom control is closely related to the depth control. As shown in Figure 5.19, it allows a portion of the image to be selected by the user for magnification. When the zoom is activated, this area is expanded and becomes the entire image.

The obvious advantages are that only the tissues of interest are being displayed and the increased magnification may allow small structures to be seen better.

Another advantage is that the zoomed image is stored using the entire image memory (i.e. all of its pixels) and hence it will retain full resolution as it is magnified.

This is in contrast to the other form of zoom known as "post-processing zoom"; this will be discussed shortly.

In addition, when the image has been zoomed using this control the machine will scan using only those lines of sight that are displayed in the zoomed image. This reduction in the number of lines of sight means that the frame rate can increase further.

Thus, in summary, the "pre-processing" (or "write") zoom function provides a better view of the tissues of interest (particularly where a small region such as the fetal heart is being examined) with no loss of pixel resolution and with increased frame rate.

The persistence function takes the most recently acquired image and averages it with the previous image (or several previous images).

This has an obvious disadvantage – rapidly moving structures will be blurred. So why is it desirable? The answer is that it smooths the speckle texture in the image.

As described earlier, speckle is the result of large numbers of low-level echoes from soft tissue combining together to produce the echo signal displayed in the image. Even slight movement of the tissues (as generally occurs with respiration, for example) and/or the probe (it is quite difficult to hold the probe absolutely still) will change the speckle.

Averaging two or more images with slightly different speckle will result in a smoother overall speckle pattern. The more images that are averaged, the smoother the texture will become. Generally the user has control of the persistence function, with the ability to turn it on and off and to alter the number of images averaged. It should be off when very dynamic tissues are being imaged (e.g. in echocardiography).

Compound imaging will be described in further detail in chapter 12. The machine acquires several images. For each image the beams are steered in a slightly different direction. The machine then combines these images to produce a single "compound" image. Advantages include smoother speckle (for similar reasons to those described above for persistence) and better imaging of tissue interfaces. This is clearly a pre-processing function since it is carried out before the final image is stored and viewed.

Extended field of view (panoramic) imaging will also be discussed in detail in chapter 12. The probe is moved in a specific way and the image area is extended to create a larger field of view. (This is similar to the panorama function on some digital cameras.)

Image memory

The image memory is simply a part of the ultrasound machine's digital memory that is used to store the image and make it available for display.

It is virtually identical in its operation to the storage of an image in a digital camera. It consists of a number of rows and columns of digital memory locations, as shown in Figures 5.21 and 5.22. Each location (a "pixel" or picture cell) stores a digital number which determines the shade of grey displayed at the corresponding point in the image.

The number of "bits" (binary digits) determines the number of different grey scale levels that can be displayed. For example, 8 bits will provide 256 different levels while 12 bits will provide 4,096 levels. The dynamic range of the display will be 24 dB for 8 bits and 36 dB for 12 bits.

As with a digital camera, the number of pixels must be sufficient that the image looks smooth and is not "pixellated". A common size is 1024 pixels wide by 768 pixels high, giving a total of 786,432 pixels.

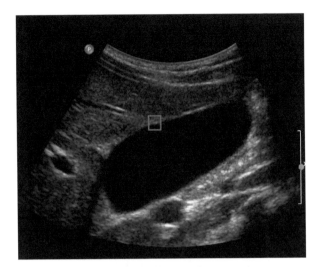

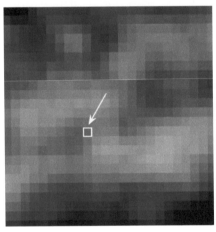

Figure 5.21 A small part of the ultrasound image on top (indicated by the box) has been magnified (bottom) to show the pixels. An individual pixel (indicated by the box) is a rectangle with its grey scale level specified by the number stored in the corresponding pixel location in the image memory.

distance along probe

depth

Figure 5.22 The image memory consists of a rectangular array of rows and columns. Each individual memory location corresponds to a pixel in the image.

An extremely useful function is the cineloop.

The machine actually contains a large number of identical image memories as shown in Figure 5.23, allowing it to retain the last 100 to 200 images. When the freeze button is pressed, imaging ceases and these images are held. The user can then move back and forward through the previous few seconds of stored images to find a specific individual image.

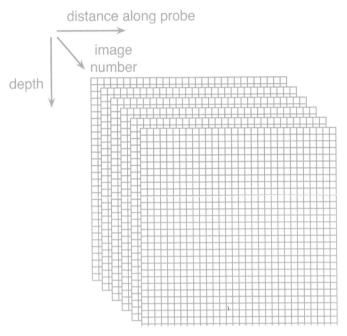

Figure 5.23 The machine contains a series of image memories. These are used to retain the previous 100 - 200 images for review using the "cineloop" function.

Post-processing

As Figure 5.17 indicates, post-processing functions are applied to the stored image as it is being read out of the image memory for display. Since these functions do not alter the stored image, their effects are reversible.

They include:

- post-processing ("read") zoom
- colour mapping
- post-processing curves
- measurements

Post-processing (or "read") zoom offers an alternative to the pre-processing zoom discussed earlier. With this zoom, a portion of the stored image is selected and expanded to fill the entire image display area on the screen.

Note that this is a function applied to a stored (frozen) image. The machine's scanning is therefore unaffected, and hence there is no beneficial impact on frame rate.

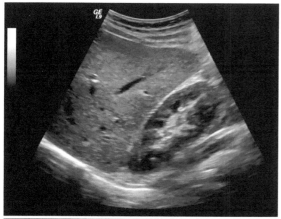

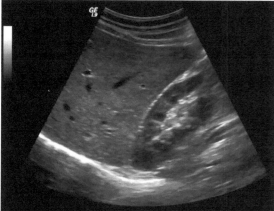

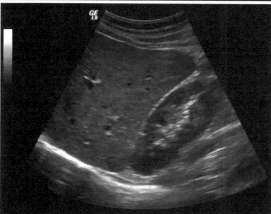

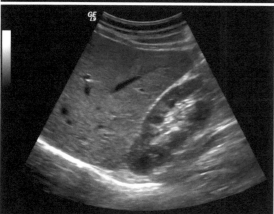

Figure 5.24 Examples of colour-mapped images. A liver image is shown here using four different colour maps.

While this zoom mode is convenient (since it can be turned on and off without altering the stored image) it has a major disadvantage. Since only part of the stored image is being displayed, it will be more pixellated in appearance because it has fewer pixels than the un-zoomed image. (Recall that an advantage of the pre-processing zoom is that the zoomed image is stored using all the pixels in the image memory.)

> *In summary, post-processing zoom is a convenient aid to viewing a stored image, but it degrades the image due to the reduced number of pixels and has no advantage with regard to frame rate. Pre-processing zoom is therefore preferred whenever possible.*

Some users find that they can better appreciate subtle variations in echogenicity if the image is displayed using colour mapping (or "B-colour"). Instead of using the standard range of grey scale values from black to white, a colour scale is used. Some examples are shown in Figure 5.24.

Another tool that is available in some machines is post-processing curves. These function in much the same way as the compression curve, determining precisely what shade of grey to use for each echo. Note that this control can do no more than fine-tune the image. It cannot correct for an inappropriate choice of compression, for example.

A very important post-processing function is measurement. Ultrasound machines allow the user to measure distances (e.g. the femur length in a fetal scan), circumferences (e.g. the abdominal circumference of a fetus), areas (e.g. the cross-sectional area of the left ventricle at a specific point in the heart cycle) and volumes (e.g. of a cyst).

It is important to recognise that while these measurements may be displayed on the screen with three-figure precision (see Figure 5.25) they are unlikely to be this accurate.

Artifacts (which will be discussed in chapter 6) cause blurring of tissue interfaces and lead to inaccuracy in the placement of the measurement calipers on the screen. It is not uncommon to find variations in measurements from the same image of up to 5% between individual sonographers. Figure 5.26 highlights this issue, with a distance measurement in a standard test object (an ultrasound phantom) being inaccurate due to the lateral smearing of the image caused by the beamwidth (as discussed in chapter 4).

Since there is likely to be significant variation between individuals in how they make measurements, detailed guidelines and protocols have been developed for critical application areas (such as early fetal measurements) in an effort to improve accuracy and repeatability.

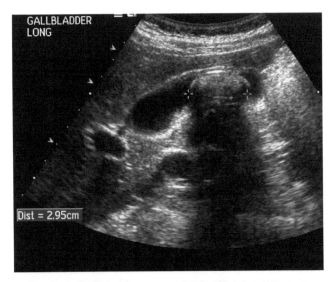

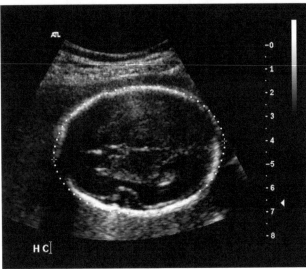

Figure 5.25 Distance measurement (top) and circumference and area measurement (bottom).

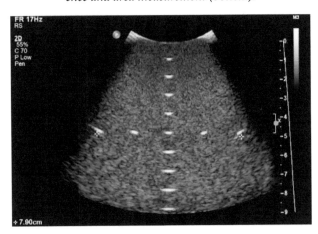

Figure 5.26 Distance measurement in an ultrasound phantom. The true distance between the point targets at the right and left edges of the image is 8.0 cm. The error in the measured distance of 7.9 cm is due to difficulty in identifying just where to place the measurement calipers.

Display

The display used by an ultrasound machine is essentially a high quality computer display. It can be expected to be stable and reliable and should require little or no adjustment or calibration.

Image storage and recording

Since the ultrasound image is digital in format, a range of options are generally available for recording and storing images.

These include:

- storage (usually short-term) within the machine's digital memory
- storage on a network, allowing them to be read and reported from a workstation elsewhere on the network
- on a CD, DVD, hard disk or other removable digital storage device
- as a hard-copy record on film or paper
- as a video (i.e. TV) format recording on DVD

Suggested activities

1. Experiment with the controls covered in this section:
   - depth
   - pre-processing zoom
   - post-processing zoom
   - persistence
   - colour mapping (B-colour)
   - cineloop
   - post-processing curves
   - measurements

2. Note the effect of persistence on the smoothness of the soft tissue texture (speckle).

3. Note the effect of the depth control and pre-processing zoom on the frame rate.

4. Compare the image quality for pre- and post-processing zoom.

5. Measure both distance and area on a structure in an image. Repeat the placement of the calipers a number of times and see if you get exactly the same value each time. Ask a colleague to measure the same structure in the same image and see if they get the same value.

Chapter 6

Image artifacts

Introductory comments

In the preceding chapters a number of artifacts commonly seen in ultrasound images have been mentioned. In this chapter we will review image artifacts more systematically. We will discuss their appearances, why they occur and typical clinical situations where they are likely to be encountered. In chapter 8 we will look at Doppler artifacts.

First, what do we mean by the term "artifact"? An artifact is any appearance in an image that does not accurately represent the anatomy that is being scanned. Tissues may be missing from the image or distorted or misplaced, or they may be misrepresented (e.g. too bright or too dark). There may also be appearances in the image that do not correspond to real tissues.

Why do artifacts occur? Broadly speaking there are four possible causes:

(a) the ultrasound is not behaving as the machine assumes (causing "acoustic artifacts");

(b) one or more equipment settings are inappropriate;

(c) the equipment is faulty;

(d) electrical interference is causing visible effects in the image.

Artifacts are common in ultrasound images, and it is important to be able to recognise them. Once an artifact is recognised it can often be ignored on the grounds that it is unlikely to cause a misdiagnosis or have any negative impact on the examination. In some cases, artifacts are themselves useful diagnostic signs, providing additional information about tissues and/or helping to highlight tissues of interest.

However, sometimes artifacts can be misleading, in which case it is particularly important that they be recognised and minimised (or eliminated if possible). A number of approaches have been taken in different textbooks to classifying artifacts. We will take a simple approach in this chapter, dealing first with "acoustic artifacts" and then with artifacts caused by equipment problems and electrical interference.

Suggested activities

1. Examine a number of images and look for any appearances that you think might be artifacts. See if you can guess what might cause these and consider whether they could lead to misdiagnosis.

2. When you are scanning, watch for likely artifacts. When you identify something that you suspect is an artifact, move the probe slightly (e.g. press it into the patient, tilt or rotate it). Watch the image and see whether the suspected artifact moves in the same way as the patient's tissues.

Imaging assumptions

What assumptions does the ultrasound machine make when it converts echo information into an image?

1. *The transmitted ultrasound beam is a narrow straight line.* This is the implicit assumption behind the fact that the machine places all echoes on a "line of sight" in the image that corresponds to the centre line of the ultrasound beam.

2. *The ultrasound travels along this straight line and does not deviate from it.* We have seen that this is not true if, for example, the beam is refracted.

3. *The ultrasound always travels directly from the transducer to a given reflector (or scatterer) and the echo from that object travels directly back to the transducer.* You can see that this assumption is required for the machine to calculate the depth of each object in the image from the arrival time of its echo.

4. *The propagation speed of the ultrasound is 1540 m/sec in all tissues.* This is not true – this is an average value for typical soft tissue.

5. *The attenuation is the same in all the tissues being imaged.* Again, this is not true.

6. *All echoes detected by the transducer are due to the most recent transmit pulse.* We have seen that the

machine attempts to ensure that this is true by using a PRF that takes into account the depth of penetration.

While it is possible to organise the discussion of artifacts around this list of assumptions, we will not do this. One reason is that some artifacts are the result of more than one of these assumptions being violated.

Instead we will categorise image artifacts broadly as acoustic or equipment-related.

We will then break acoustic artifacts up into four subcategories:

- attenuation artifacts;
- depth artifacts;
- beam dimension artifacts;
- beam path artifacts.

Attenuation artifacts

These are particularly common artifacts, and you will learn to recognise them so easily that you will virtually ignore them except when they can serve a useful purpose.

Table 6.1 lists typical attenuation coefficient values for a number of tissues and for air.

Material	α (dB/cm/MHz)
blood	0.15
fat	0.6
brain	0.45
breast	0.55
liver	0.5
muscle	1.4 (along fibres) 3.3 (across fibres)
bone	10
lung	40

Table 6.1 Typical attenuation coefficient values.

It is clear that the attenuation varies significantly.

Liquids such as blood have very low attenuation while fibrous tissue has a relatively high attenuation.

Bone and air (and other materials with very different acoustic impedance to soft tissue) reflect much of the energy that strikes them, allowing only a small fraction to travel into deeper tissues and hence attenuating the ultrasound strongly.

You will remember that the machine's TGC function corrects for the average value for soft tissue (around 0.5 dB/cm/MHz).

You will also remember that the user can adjust the TGC sliders to compensate for variations in the attenuation (e.g. between amniotic fluid and fetal tissues).

However, when there are relatively small localised regions with different attenuation to the surrounding tissues, the TGC cannot correct for this, and artifacts can occur.

Shadowing

"Shadowing" is the term used to describe a darkened line cast behind (i.e. deep to) a region whose tissues cause greater attenuation than the surrounding tissues.

The increased attenuation means that the transmitted intensity beyond the region is reduced compared to the intensity at the same depth elsewhere in the image (see Figure 6.1). Echoes coming from this area will therefore be lower in amplitude than they would otherwise be.

Furthermore, these echoes will pass through the highly attenuating tissue on their way back to the transducer, again being attenuated more than echoes elsewhere in the image.

As Figures 6.1 shows, the result will be a darkened area (due to the reduced echo amplitude) in the region behind the highly attenuating tissue. Note that the shadow will always be in the direction of the ultrasound beam.

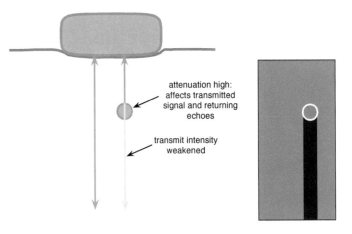

Figure 6.1 (Left) Both the transmitted ultrasound and the returning echoes are attenuated more than usual as they pass through the highly attenuating region. As a consequence the echoes from tissues deep to the region are abnormally low, creating a shadow in the image (right).

If the attenuation is only moderately increased compared with the rest of the tissues, the shadowed region may still show echoes from deeper tissues, but reduced in amplitude.

If the attenuation is very high, however, there may be no detectable echoes from the deeper tissues at all. The shadowed region may then be echo-free (a "clean" shadow) or it may contain artifactual echoes, in which case it is termed a "dirty" shadow.

Common situations where shadowing occurs are where there are gallstones in the region being imaged or where bones are present (e.g. in third trimester fetal scans). Figure 6.2 is a typical example of shadowing.

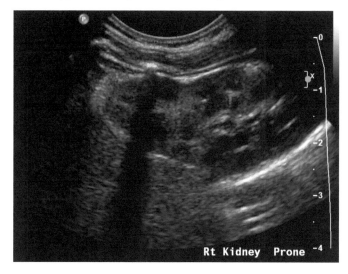

Figure 6.2 Shadowing caused by a strongly echogenic structure.

Artifacts can be useful precisely because they provide different information about the patient's tissues to what is usually imaged – the reflectivity or "echogenicity" of the tissues. Thus shadowing highlights regions with substantially higher attenuation than the surrounding tissues. For example, it can be very useful as a way to locate gallstones.

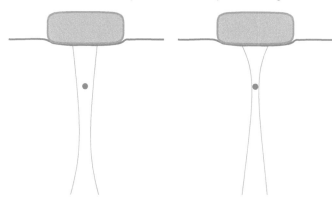

Figure 6.3 (Left) If the beam is wide relative to an attenuating object, only a small fraction of its energy will be removed and the shadowing effect will be minimal. (Right) Conversely, if the object is at focus it will block more of the energy in the beam and the shadowing will be more evident in the image.

There is an important practical consideration, however. Consider a small highly attenuating object (see Figure 6.3). It should be clear from this diagram that the beam should be made as narrow as possible at the depth where the gallstone is located. This will maximise the amount of energy removed from the beam by the gallstone and so it will maximise the shadowing effect.

It is therefore important that the transmit focus is set at the depth where the attenuating object is known (or suspected) to be located, as shown in Figure 6.4.

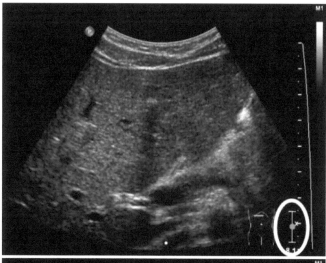

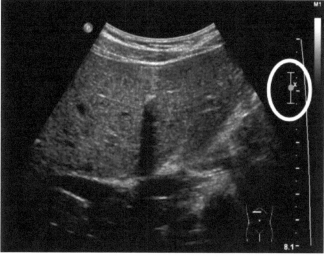

Figure 6.4 (Top) When the focus (circled) is set much deeper than the shadowing object then the shadow is poorly seen. (Bottom) With the focus placed at the same depth as the object the shadow is clearer.

Enhancement

"Enhancement" is a closely related artifact. It occurs when a region has *lower* attenuation than the surrounding tissues. The result is a brightened area behind that region, the opposite of a shadow (see Figure 6.5).

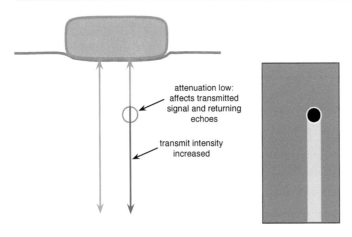

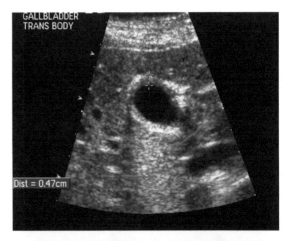

Figure 6.5 Enhancement occurs when a region with low attenuation lies in the path of the ultrasound. This attenuates the transmitted ultrasound (and the returning echo) less than would be the case in its absence. The echoes deep to the region are therefore brighter than expected.

A typical example is when a liquid-filled structure is imaged (e.g. a cyst, or the gallbladder). Most liquids have substantially lower attenuation than soft tissue, and therefore cause enhancement.

Like attenuation, enhancement can be a very useful diagnostic sign. As with shadowing, when a small object is causing enhancement (e.g. a small cyst), enhancement will be maximised when the beam is focussed at the depth of the object.

Edge shadowing

"Edge shadowing" (sometimes called "refractive edge shadowing") is another type of shadowing.

The cause is quite different to that described above, as Figure 6.7 shows. Edge shadowing occurs when the ultrasound beam strikes the edge of a circular structure (e.g. a cyst or a blood vessel in cross-section). A combination of reflection and refraction occurs, causing the ultrasound beam to be deflected and broadened (i.e. defocussed).

As explained in chapter 4, there is an inverse relationship between the width of the beam and the intensity. The broadening of the beam due to its interaction with the edge of the circular structure therefore leads to a reduction in beam intensity. As a consequence, echoes from the tissues beyond the edges of the circular structure will be reduced in amplitude, leading to shadowing.

Since the ultrasound machine is unaware that the beam has been deflected, these echoes will be displayed in the image as though they have come from the tissues where the beam would have travelled if it had not been deflected (see Figures 6.7 and 6.8).

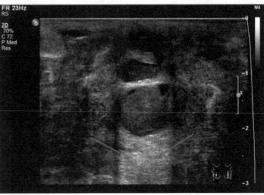

Figure 6.6. (Top) Enhancement due to the low attenuation of ultrasound by the gallbladder (arrows). (Bottom) Enhancement caused by an abscess in the breast, demonstrating that not all enhancement is caused by echo free regions (arrows).

We therefore have two effects: (a) the echoes are reduced in amplitude, and (b) they are displaced since the beam has not travelled in a straight line but the machine assumes that it has.

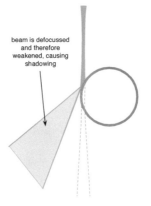
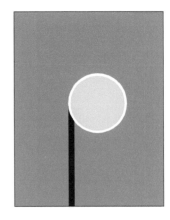

Figure 6.7 Most of the energy in the ultrasound beam is deflected from the edge of the circular object. This spreads the beam out (i.e. defocusses it) which reduces the beam intensity. The weak echoes coming from the defocussed beam are displayed as if the beam had continued in a straight line, causing edge shadowing.

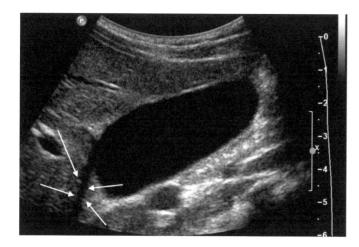

Figure 6.8 (a) Edge shadowing (arrows) caused by the liquid-filled gallbladder.

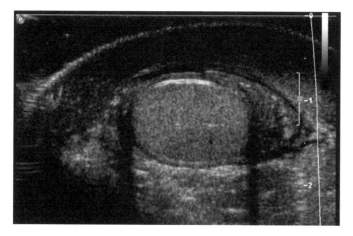

Figure 6.8 (b) Edge shadowing caused by a testis, showing that a variety of circular structures can cause edge shadowing and that they need not be perfectly circular.

Edge shadowing is very common in ultrasound images. It generally is of little value diagnostically, and it is therefore largely ignored.

Suggested activities

1. Watch for examples of shadowing and enhancement as you scan. Try to identify the structure causing each artifact. Would you expect it to have higher (or lower) attenuation than average tissue?

2. View ultrasound images of circular structures (e.g. blood vessels in cross-section) and look for edge shadowing.

3. Move the probe and see if the direction of the shadows changes as the scanning direction changes.

Depth artifacts

A number of artifacts lead to incorrect display of the depth of tissues. These include propagation speed, reverberation, comet-tail and ring-down artifacts. (Range ambiguity is yet another depth artifact, but it is only likely to be encountered in connection with pulsed Doppler, so it will be discussed with other Doppler artifacts in chapter 8.)

Propagation speed artifact

As mentioned above, when the machine calculates the depth at which to display each echo in the image it assumes that the propagation speed of sound is 1540 m/sec in all tissues. In reality the propagation speed varies somewhat from one tissue type to another, as shown in Table 6.2. Fat, for example, has a significantly lower propagation speed.

Material	c (m/sec)
blood	1575
fat	1450
brain	1560
breast	1430 - 1570
liver	1570
muscle	1530 - 1630
bone	2000 - 4000
lung	650

Table 6.2 Typical propagation speed values.

If the ultrasound travels through a significant amount of tissue with propagation speed different to 1540 m/sec, the depth at which echoes will be displayed will be incorrect.

Consider the situation shown in Figure 6.9, where the ultrasound travels through a fatty region in the liver. Both the transmitted ultrasound and the echoes returning from tissues deep to the region will be slowed down while they are travelling through it.

Echoes from tissues beyond the fatty region will therefore arrive at the transducer later than they would if the fatty region was absent, and so they will be displayed deeper than they should be.

Conversely, if the ultrasound passes through a region with propagation speed higher than 1540 m/sec then echoes from deeper tissues will arrive more quickly than if the speed in the region had been 1540 m/sec and so the tissues will be displayed more superficially than their true position.

In both cases the displacement of tissues in depth will only occur for the tissues in line with the region which has a different propagation speed and deep to it.

A typical appearance is therefore as shown in Figure 6.9, where a linear structure (e.g. the diaphragm as imaged through the liver) will appear to be displaced locally in the area behind the region with different propagation speed.

A clinical example is shown in Figure 6.10.

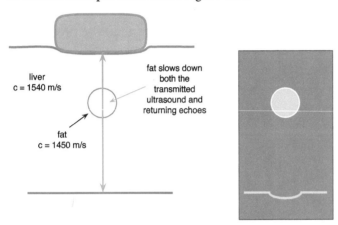

Figure 6.9 A region with lower propagation speed (e.g. a fatty region within a liver) will slow down both the transmitted ultrasound and returning echoes, causing the machine to display structures which are deep to the region as being farther away than their true position.

Reverberation artifact

Reverberation artifacts cause tissue structures to be displayed multiple times at equally spaced depths in the image.

When we talk about the acoustics of a concert hall, the term "reverberation" is used to describe the effect of sound reflecting back and forth between parallel surfaces (e.g. the floor and ceiling of the hall, or across the width of the hall between the side walls). Indeed, without reverberation the hall would be said to have a very "dead" sound.

In ultrasound, the term means the same thing – it describes the reflection of ultrasound repeatedly back and forth between two parallel surfaces, as shown in Figure 6.11.

Clearly this will happen only if the surfaces have relatively large reflection coefficients. Examples include the interface between the transducer and skin surface (particularly if there is not sufficient coupling gel), tissue/bone interfaces, calcified structures, fibrous and air-filled structures.

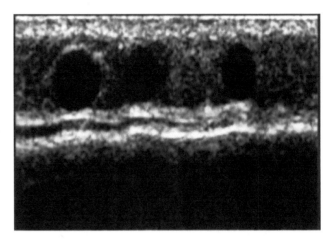

Figure 6.10 The slightly higher propagation speed in these varicose veins makes the tibial plateau appear falsely wavy in this image.

As Figure 6.11 shows, a series of echoes will return to the transducer. The image will therefore show the reflecting surfaces in their true position and then replicated a number of times, with the spacing between the echoes being equal to the distance between the two reflecting surfaces.

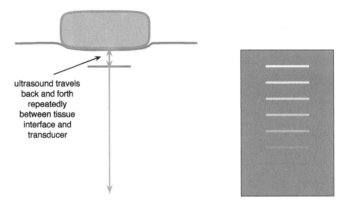

Figure 6.11(a) When ultrasound is reflected back and forth between a tissue interface and the transducer face a series of equally spaced echoes will be seen, progressively weakening in brightness with depth.

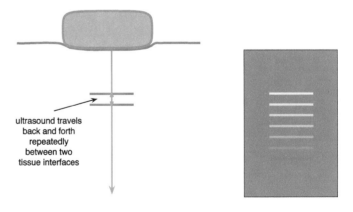

Figure 6.11(b) A similar appearance is seen when the ultrasound reverberates between two tissue layers.

If soft tissue lies between the reflecting interfaces, it too will be duplicated in the image (see Figure 6.12).

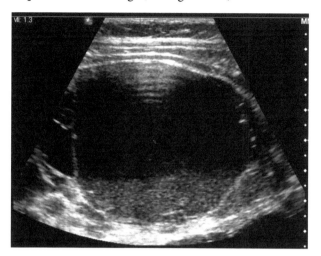

Figure 6.12 (a) Reverberation has caused a series of parallel echoes to appear in the superficial portion of a haemorrhagic renal cyst.

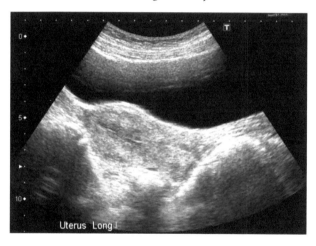

Figure 6.12 (b) In this image, reverberation has caused soft tissue echoes to be duplicated and appear inside the urinary bladder.

Ring-down artifact

A special case of reverberation occurs when the reflectors are small gas bubbles (e.g. as commonly found in the gastrointestinal tract). As Figure 6.13 shows, multiple echoes will return to the transducer as the ultrasound reverberates back and forth among the gas bubbles.

If the gas bubbles are in liquid (which is usually the case) there will be very little attenuation, and so the sequence of echoes returning to the transducer will remain strong over time. Since the reflection of ultrasound by gas bubbles is highly efficient (i.e. very little energy is lost during reflection) the result is a bright line of echoes deep to the bubbles, as shown in Figure 6.14.

This is known as the ring-down artifact.

Note that discrete echoes from individual bubbles cannot be identified, with the artifact instead being a relatively continuous line of bright echoes.

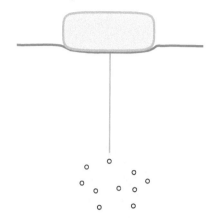

Figure 6.13 Ultrasound reflects between multiple gas bubbles, creating a continuous series of echoes returning to the transducer. The result is a bright echo extending in depth from the gas bubbles along the beam direction.

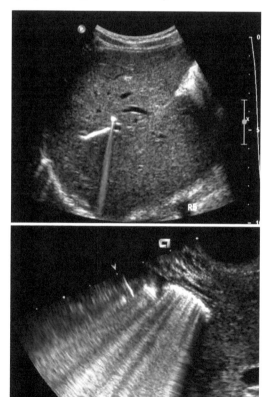

Figure 6.14 Two examples of ring-down artifact. (Top) A typical example due to gas in the liver. (Bottom) A dramatic example due to gas-filled bowel.

In some texts the ring-down artifact is said to be caused by resonant vibration of the bubbles. This has been questioned in recent times, and it is believed that resonance is not necessary for the formation of the artifact. If resonance does occur, it would be expected to intensify the effect.

Comet-tail artifact

Another closely-related type of reverberation artifact is the comet-tail artifact.

As Figure 6.15 shows, this is similar to the ring-down artifact but it is shorter-lived and hence it is seen as a relatively short "tail" extending into the tissues, tapering and fading in a manner similar to the typical "tail" of a comet.

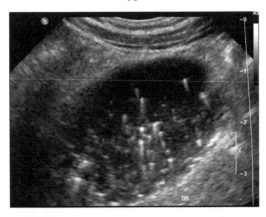

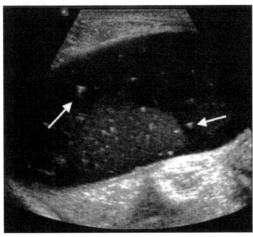

Figure 6.15 (Top) Relatively prominent comet-tail artifacts in a gallbladder filled with "sludge". (Bottom) A second example where the comet-tails are subtler (in part because the gain is set lower in this scan).

Generally this artifact is caused by small calcifications. These are strong reflectors of ultrasound, like gas bubbles. As the ultrasound reverberates between a group of calcifications it produces a series of echoes, just as with the ring-down artifact. However, there is a major difference between ring-down and comet-tail artifacts.

The reflection of ultrasound by gas bubbles is highly efficient, so little energy is lost in the process and the artifact generally extends at full brightness to the maximum depth displayed.

In contrast, the reflection of ultrasound by calcium causes significant loss of energy and hence with reverberation the echoes quickly reduce in amplitude and so the artifact fades from the image with depth.

Comet-tail artifact can also be caused by foreign bodies such as biopsy needles.

Suggested activities

1. As you scan in the abdomen, look for examples of reverberation, ring-down and comet-tail artifact.

2. Try to identify the likely source of the artifact. Move the transducer slightly, both by translation over the patient's skin and by pressing it more firmly into the patient, and note the effect on the artifact.

Beam dimension artifacts

Beamwidth artifact

In chapter 4 there is a description of the effect of the transducer's beamwidth on the ultrasound image. In brief, every point in the image is smeared laterally by an amount equal to the beamwidth (see Figure 6.16).

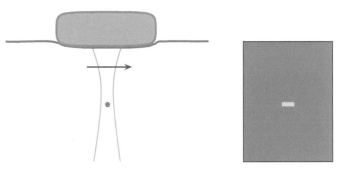

Figure 6.16 As the ultrasound beam scans from left to right, it displays a point multiple times at slightly different positions, creating a line in the image perpendicular to the beam direction and equal to the beamwidth in size.

If a tissue interface is scanned, as shown in Figures 6.17, 6.18 and 6.19, every point on the interface will be smeared in this way.

If the interface is between soft tissue and liquid (e.g. a heart wall or the wall of a cyst) the smearing will be visible in the image as fuzziness of the boundary.

Figures 6.17 and 6.18 show how beamwidth artifact depends on the orientation of the interface relative to the beam. When the incidence is perpendicular (as shown in Figure 6.18) the beamwidth artifact is eliminated. It follows that when you are imaging fine structures (e.g. the membranes encountered in nuchal translucency scans) you should always attempt to keep the ultrasound beam perpendicular to the interface. Not only will this eliminate beamwidth artifact but it will also maximise the echo strength as discussed earlier.

Figures 6.19 and 6.20 show the effect of beamwidth artifact when a curved tissue interface is scanned. Again note that the image of the interface will be fuzzy except where the beam strikes it at 90°.

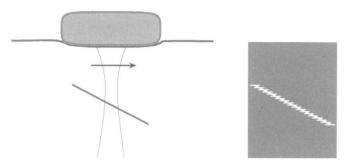

Figure 6.17 A tissue interface will be "fuzzy" in the image due to beamwidth artifact.

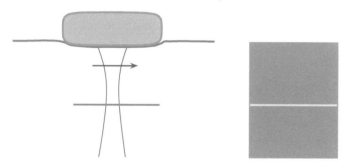

Figure 6.18 If the tissue interface is imaged at perpendicular incidence (i.e. the beam strikes the interface at 90°) the fuzziness is not visible and it does not degrade the image.

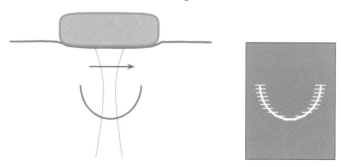

Figure 6.19 Beamwidth artifact associated with a curved tissue interface.

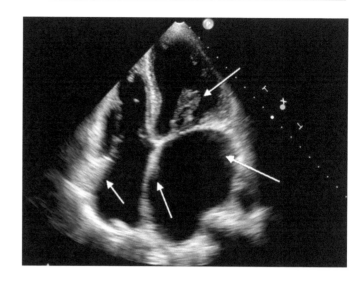

Figure 6.20 Beamwidth artifact in the heart. The upper arrow shows a lesion. The three lower arrows highlight areas where beamwidth artifact is very evident. Note how the fuzziness tends to increase with depth since the beamwidth increases with depth.

Sidelobe artifact

Chapter 4 also introduced the concept of sidelobes.

These are unwanted additional beams symmetrically positioned either side of the main beam (see Figure 6.21). They are always present, although fortunately they are considerably weaker than the main beam.

Nevertheless, when a strong reflector is present in a sidelobe it can generate a detectable echo, in which case the echo will be displayed as though it had come from the main beam (see Figure 6.21).

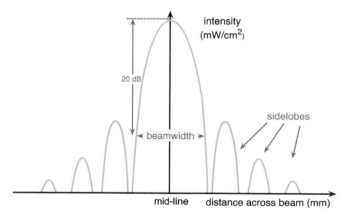

Figure 6.21 (a) A graph of the intensity distribution across the beam showing the sidelobes either side of the main beam. The strongest sidelobe is the one nearest to the main beam.

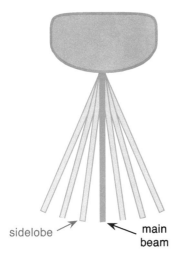

Figure 6.21 (b) The sidelobes are symmetrically positioned to left and right of the main beam.

As Figure 6.22 shows, when the main beam scans from left to right to acquire a full image, a reflector will be imaged in its true location (by the main beam) and also to the left and right of its true position (by the sidelobes).

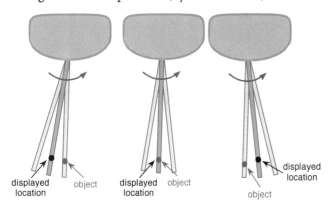

Figure 6.22 (a) As the machine scans the main beam from left to right, the sidelobes will also be scanned. For simplicity only the strongest sidelobes are shown here.

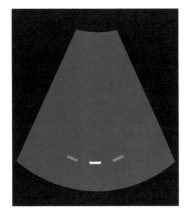

Figure 6.22 (b) Strong reflectors will therefore be displayed in multiple positions in the image.

Figure 6.23 shows a clinical example of sidelobe artifact.

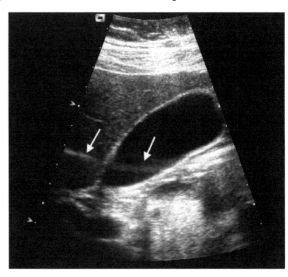

Figure 6.23 Example of a sidelobe artifact (arrows). Strong echoes caused by duodenal gas have been replicated (with reduced intensity) to the left and right of the gas. The artifact is most readily seen in the gallbladder.

Slice thickness artifact

In chapter 4 we also discussed slice thickness and its effect on image quality.

Figures 6.24, 6.25 and 6.26 illustrate the concept of slice thickness.

Recall that the thickness is determined by how well (or poorly) the beam is focussed in the direction across the width of the transducer.

Most transducers achieve this focussing using a lens (as shown in Figure 6.24), although the newer "matrix" transducers allow electronic focussing in this dimension too (as discussed in chapter 4).

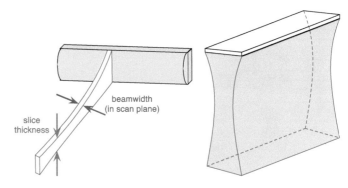

Figure 6.24 (Left) The beam is focussed within the scan plane (by electronic focussing) and in the slice thickness direction (by a lens). (Right) As the beam scans along the length of the transducer it acquires echoes from a volume.

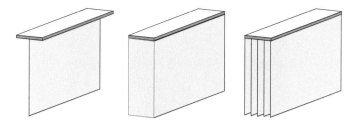

Figure 6.25 (Left) An ideal thin scan plane. (Centre) In reality the scan plane is thick, as shown here; for simplicity it is shown as having uniform slice thickness. (Right) It is convenient to consider the scan as being the sum of a number of thin scan planes as shown.

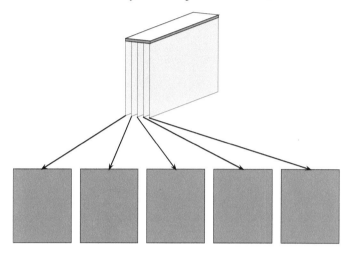

Figure 6.26 The overall image obtained from the real scan plane can be thought of as the sum of the images obtained from each of the idealised thin scan planes.

Many structures can be scanned in such a way that the effect of slice thickness on the image is minimal.

Figure 6.27 shows an example, where the probe has been positioned so that the axis of a vessel is perpendicular to the scan plane. All of the imaginary thin slices contain identical images and so their sum, too, shows a clean circular cross-section of the vessel. Compare this with the situation shown in Figure 6.28, where the vessel is at an angle to the scan plane.

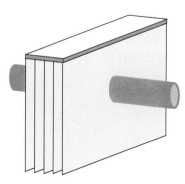

Figure 6.27 (a) A short axis scan of a vessel.

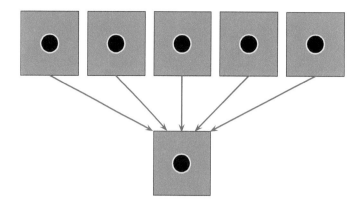

Figure 6.27 (b) Since the vessel is perpendicular to the scan plane, each of the images from the thin slices is the same. When they are added together the result is a clean circular image of the vessel with no slice thickness artifact.

The first thing to notice is that the cross-sectional view of the vessel is no longer circular, but elliptical due to the angle.

Secondly, the image will be fuzzy. This happens because the vessel is in a slightly different position in each of the idealised thin slices and so it becomes fuzzy when they are combined together.

A clinical example is shown in Figure 6.29.

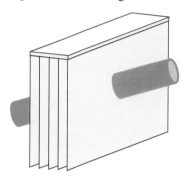

Figure 6.28 (a) A vessel imaged at an angle. It will appear elliptical in the image due to the oblique angle.

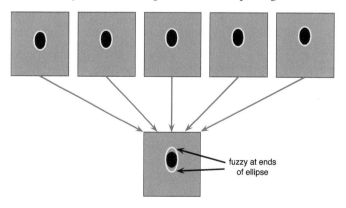

Figure 6.28 (b) The vessel is at a different position in each of the thin slices and so the resultant image is fuzzy when they are combined.

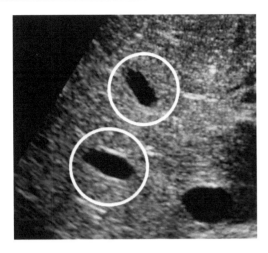

Figure 6.29 The circled vessels in this liver scan are elliptical because they are at an oblique angle to the scan plane. They are well-defined across their diameters but the ends of the ellipses are fuzzy due to slice thickness artifact.

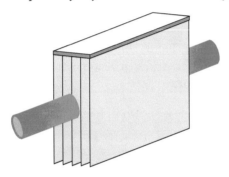

Figure 6.30 (a) A long axis scan of a vessel.

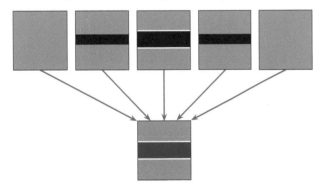

Figure 6.30 (b) Not all of the thin slices pass through the vessel, and so it is not displayed in all of them. Furthermore, only one slice passes through the centre of the vessel, and so only it shows the true vessel diameter. The result is that the vessel contains echoes from adjacent tissues at the same depth.

What is the effect of slice thickness if the scan plane is aligned with the long axis of a vessel? Figures 6.30 and 6.31 show that artifactual echoes from the tissues on either side of the vessel will be displayed within the vessel. An exception is when the diameter of the vessel is considerably larger than the slice thickness, but this is not common.

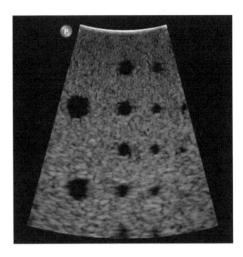

Figure 6.31 (a) Scan of an ultrasound test object containing a series of parallel "vessels". Here the vessels at all depths are free of internal echoes but beamwidth artifact is evident, especially in the deeper vessels.

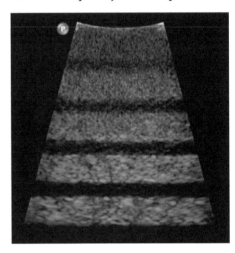

Figure 6.31 (b) In contrast, this long axis view shows internal echoes due to slice thickness artifact, especially in the superficial region where the slice thickness is larger.

Figure 6.32 shows an example where a strong reflector intrudes part-way into the slice thickness and therefore contributes to the image. Since it is only partially within the slice thickness it is not as bright in the image as it would be if it was wholly within it.

Suggested activities

1. Scan a vessel (e.g. the common carotid artery) in cross-section. Position the probe to give a circular cross-section, then tilt it to create an elliptical view. Watch for any fuzziness due to slice thickness effects.

2. Look for examples of sidelobe artifact while you are scanning. They are only likely to be visible in echo-free liquid-filled areas.

3. Watch for any partial volume effects while you scan, for example low-level tissue echoes within liquid-filled structures caused by nearby tissues.

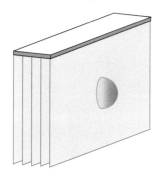

Figure 6.32 (a) An example of a situation where the partial volume effect occurs. A mass intruding part-way into the slice thickness of the scan will be weakly displayed in the image.

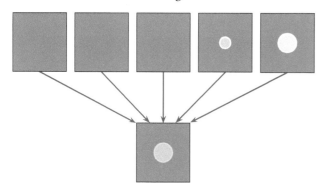

Figure 6.32 (b) The partial volume effect. A spherical mass intrudes part-way into the slice thickness. It is therefore seen in only some of the thin slices, causing it to be displayed less strongly than if it was fully within the scan plane.

Beam path artifacts

Refraction artifact

You will remember the discussion of refraction in chapter 2. It refers to the change in the direction of travel of ultrasound when it passes through an interface between two tissues with significantly different propagation speeds (see Figure 6.33).

The change of direction is more pronounced if the angle of incidence is large (i.e. well away from perpendicular incidence) and if the difference in propagation speed is large.

Conversely, if the ultrasound beam strikes an interface at perpendicular incidence there is no refraction, regardless of whether there is a difference in propagation speed between the two tissues.

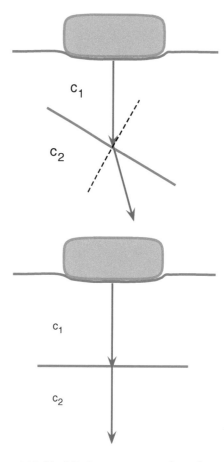

Figure 6.33 (Top) Refraction occurs when ultrasound passes through an interface between two tissues with different propagation speeds. (Bottom) An exception is when the ultrasound is at perpendicular incidence.

An important additional comment needs to be made. Snell's Law (which determines the amount of refraction) shows that ultrasound echoes can follow exactly the same path as the incident ultrasound back to the transducer. Figure 6.34 therefore shows arrows at either end of the ultrasound path.

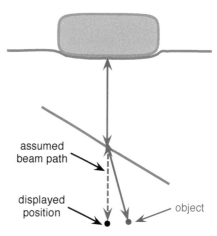

Figure 6.34 Since the machine assumes that ultrasound travels in a straight line, refraction will cause this object to be displaced in the image.

The ultrasound machine, however, assumes that the ultrasound has travelled in a straight line, and so it displays the reflecting object at a slightly different position than its true location.

The effect of refraction on the ultrasound image is usually small and generally not noticeable. However, particularly striking refraction artifacts can occur in the abdomen when a transverse scan is done with the transducer located on the patient's midline.

The rectus abdominis muscle is composed of two lens-shaped sections, as shown in Figure 6.35. This can significantly alter the direction of travel of the ultrasound, causing the image of objects deeper than the muscle to be displaced, as shown in Figure 6.36.

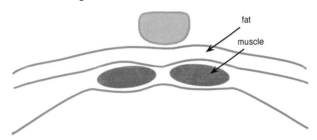

Figure 6.35 The rectus abdominis muscle takes the form of two lenses in cross-section.

Due to the symmetry of the geometry, the distortion of the image is also symmetrical. For example, a vessel (such as the superior mesenteric artery in cross-section) will be displaced to both the left and right of its true position, as shown in Figure 6.36.

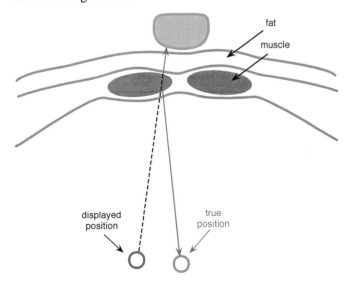

Figure 6.36 (a) As the beam scans from left to right, it is deflected as shown, producing a displaced image of the vessel to the left of its true position. (In this diagram the displacement is exaggerated for clarity.)

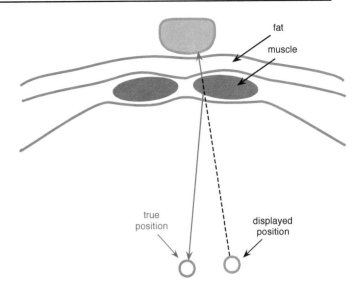

Figure 6.36 (b) As the beam continues to scan from left to right it is deflected again, producing a displaced image of the vessel to the right of its true position

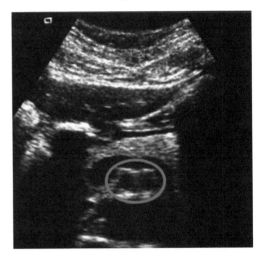

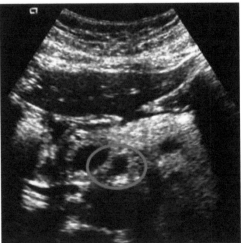

Figure 6.37 (Top) In this image the superior mesenteric artery (circled) appears to be doubled. (Bottom) Moving the transducer to one side removes the symmetry of the refraction and it is seen to be a single vessel.

The result is an apparent doubling of the vessel in the image, as shown in Figure 6.37.

Moving the probe towards the patient's left or right side (i.e. away from the midline) removes the symmetry of the geometry and it becomes clear that it is really a single vessel.

Mirror image artifact

Reflection of ultrasound was also discussed in chapter 2. A typical reflector is an interface between two tissues that have significantly different acoustic impedances (e.g. the diaphragm, which is the interface between the soft tissue in the liver and the air-filled lungs). The geometry of reflection is very simple; the incident angle is equal to the reflected angle.

Again an echo can follow exactly the same path as the incident ultrasound back to the transducer.

Since the machine assumes that the ultrasound has travelled in a straight line, it displays the reflecting object in an entirely wrong location (see Figure 6.38). As the beam scans it will therefore create an image of the tissues beyond the interface.

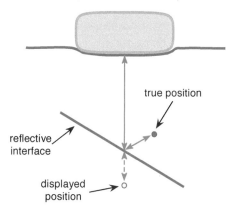

Figure 6.38 In the presence of a strongly reflective interface, tissues can be imaged by reflected ultrasound. Since the machine assumes the ultrasound has travelled in a straight line, the tissues will be displayed behind the interface, as shown. Often they will also be displayed in their true location.

This is exactly what happens with light and a mirror, and hence the artifact is known as the mirror image artifact. It is quite commonly encountered, especially when scanning the liver. An example is shown in Figure 6.39.

What happens if the reflecting interface (the "mirror") is curved? The effect is the same as when you look at yourself in a curved mirror – the artifact is distorted. An example is shown in Figure 6.40.

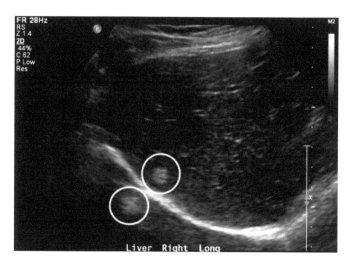

Figure 6.39 A liver lesion and its mirror image behind the diaphragm.

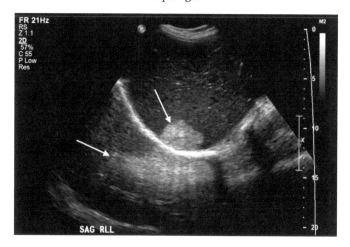

Figure 6.40 Note the distortion of this mirror image due to the curvature of the diaphragm.

Even more complicated is the situation where the "mirror" is not perpendicular to the scan plane. The geometry is shown in Figure 6.41.

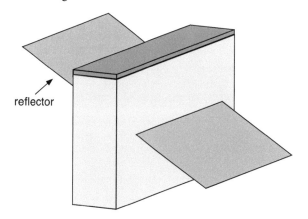

Figure 6.41 (a) A strongly reflective tissue interface passes through the scan plane at an angle.

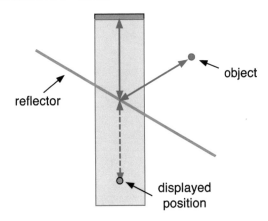

Figure 6.41 (b) An end view of the scan plane shows the ultrasound reflecting out of the scan plane and striking an object. Echoes from the object return along the same path to the transducer. Since the machine assumes the ultrasound has travelled in a straight line, the object is displayed below the reflecting interface. Note that the object will not be seen in the image in its true position, since it lies outside the scan plane.

In this case the object that appears in the mirror image lies outside the scan plane and so it will not be seen in the image in its true location, only the mirror image will be seen.

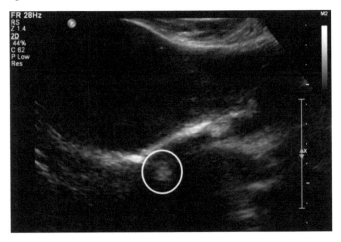

Figure 6.42 The same liver lesion as shown in Figure 6.39. However, in this case the diaphragm is not perpendicular to the scan plane and so only the mirror image is seen.

Figure 6.42 is a clinical example of a mirror image where the reflecting interface is at an angle to the scan plane, and so only the mirror image is displayed.

Suggested activities

1. Try to produce an example of the refraction artifact described above (where structures such as the mesenteric artery are doubled in transverse abdominal scans). Move the probe to the left or right from the patient's midline and note the effect on the artifact.

2. Look for examples of mirror image artifact as you scan. When you find an example analyse the image to determine what the reflecting interface is and what path the ultrasound has followed to produce the artifact.

3. Note whether the structures in a mirror image are also displayed in their true location, or whether you need to move the probe to see them. Try to obtain a scan plane such that both the true location and the mirror image are in the same image (as in Figure 6.39).

Equipment and electrical artifacts

Finally, we will discuss very briefly artifacts caused by malfunction of the machine, incorrect settings and electrical interference.

The most likely cause of equipment malfunction is damage to the probe. If a probe is dropped or bumped against a hard surface, it is possible that one or more transducer elements will cease to work. This can cause an area of drop-out or other abnormalities in the image (see Figure 6.43).

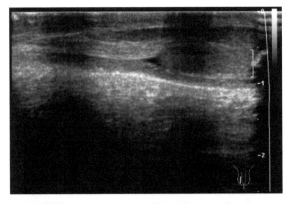

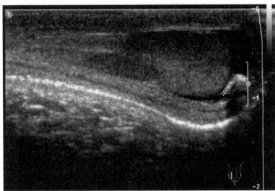

Figure 6.43 (Top) Testicular scan showing dark bands due to a transducer fault. (Bottom) A scan of the same patient with a normal probe.

Note that the drop-out will be fixed in position relative to the transducer face. As the probe scans the artifact will move with it, making it clear that it is an equipment problem rather than something relating to the patient's tissues.

In chapter 5 the major equipment controls were introduced. While the machine's presets generally provide reasonably good images, the user should always be ready to fine-tune the controls to adjust for variations in the clinical situation.

Incorrect settings can lead to misleading appearances and the potential for misdiagnosis.

For example, wrong setting of the overall gain and TGC can make some tissues appear less or more echogenic than they should be. Incorrect choice of frequency can cause dropout (if the frequency is too high) or poor resolution (if it is too low). Incorrect focus and depth settings will lead to suboptimal images and loss of detail.

The use of persistence when imaging highly dynamic tissues such as the fetal heart will cause blurring of moving tissues in the image. Incorrect dynamic range settings can alter the image appearance and can also cause loss of detail.

Electrical interference is generally not a problem except when portable equipment is being used in electrically noisy environments such as a Neonatal Intensive Care Unit. It may then produce a variety of patterns in the image.

As with equipment faults, it is easy to see by watching the image (particularly in real time) that these patterns are not related to the tissues being scanned (see Figure 6.44).

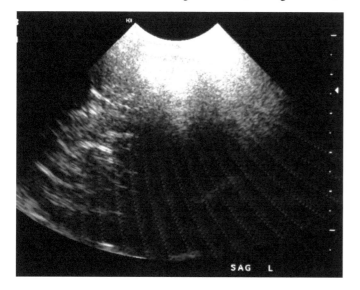

Figure 6.44 The curved lines in this image (most readily visible in the lower right-hand part of the image where the tissue image has dropped out) are due to electrical interference.

Summary

Artifacts are frequently seen in ultrasound images, particularly in fluid-filled areas and other areas with low echo levels.

Some artifacts are useful indicators of tissue properties – shadowing and enhancement indicate regions of abnormally high or low attenuation respectively, ring-down artifact usually indicates the presence of gas bubbles, comet-tail artifact is often caused by calcifications, etc.

Other artifacts have the potential to mislead and possibly cause misdiagnosis. They may also conceal useful information (think of ring-down artifact, for example).

In fact artifacts are present in every image. Every structure in the image is affected by beamwidth artifact, for example. Aside from the recognisable artifacts referred to above, what is the impact of this?

It can be useful to think of the image as being composed of an "ideal" ultrasound image which then has artifacts added to it. Clearly the fewer artifacts there are the more readily subtle variations in tissue echogenicity and texture can be seen. This will be discussed in chapter 10 under the heading "contrast resolution". Some of the newer imaging modes (harmonics and compound scanning, for example) can substantially reduce artifacts, and this explains why they are so widely used.

Artifacts are often a product of the geometric arrangement of the probe and tissues (think of reverberation, for example). Moving or angling the probe will therefore modify (or even eliminate) most artifacts. This is useful both as a way to identify the appearances in an image as artifacts and as a means to reduce or eliminate them.

Finally, artifacts vary greatly in their appearance and can appear quite unexpectedly at times – you need to be actively thinking and analysing your images at all times as you scan!

Chapter 7

Doppler ultrasound

The Doppler effect and its applications in ultrasound

Doppler ultrasound began as a specialised technique used only in cardiac and vascular applications, but it has since proved to be broadly useful. Now the various Doppler modes – pulsed Doppler, colour Doppler and continuous wave Doppler – are widely used.

Doppler differs from imaging in an important way. Imaging provides information primarily about structure, whereas Doppler is used to get information about function (blood flow and tissue motion).

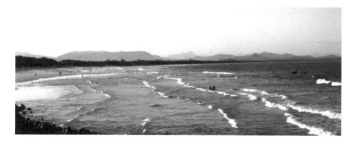

Figure 7.1

What do we mean by the Doppler effect? Imagine yourself standing in the water at the beach shown in Figure 7.1. If you stand still, 12 waves pass by you each minute and so you say the waves have a frequency of 12/60 = 0.20 Hz. Now imagine that you walk directly away from the beach and towards the oncoming waves. Because you are moving, you now see 15 waves each minute, so you say that the frequency is 15/60 = 0.25 Hz. You then turn around and walk directly towards the beach. Just 9 waves now pass you every minute, since you and the waves are travelling in the same direction, so you say the frequency is 9/60 = 0.15 Hz.

This is an example of the Doppler effect. The frequency of the ocean waves appears to change depending on whether you are stationary or moving.

It increases if you are moving towards the waves and decreases if you are moving in the same direction that they are travelling.

This effect occurs with all types of wave energy (radio waves, light, sound etc). When there is motion of either the source or the receiver, the observed frequency changes. The amount by which the frequency changes is termed the Doppler shift. Thus in the above example the Doppler shift is 0.05 Hz.

The amount of Doppler shift is determined by how fast the movement is.

By measuring the Doppler shift we can therefore get information about the speed of movement of objects. (This is the basis of police radar for example.)

Now let us consider how Doppler ultrasound is used to obtain information about flowing blood, since this is its main application.

When ultrasound is reflected by moving blood, the echoes returning to the probe will have a slightly different frequency than the frequency that was transmitted due to the Doppler shift. This has no noticeable effect on the grey scale image. However, when the machine is operating in Doppler mode it detects the Doppler shift and displays it, providing information about the blood flow velocity.

For example (see Figure 7.2), if 5 MHz ultrasound is reflected by blood which is travelling towards the probe at a speed of 100 cm/sec the returning echo will have a frequency of 5.0065 MHz. The frequency of the echo has thus increased by 6.5 kHz and so the Doppler shift is 6.5 kHz.

If the blood was moving away from the probe at the same speed, the received echo would have a frequency of 4.9935 MHz, and so the frequency would have decreased by the same Doppler shift amount (i.e. 6.5 kHz).

How does the Doppler shift relate to the blood velocity? As we would expect, it is directly proportional to it. The faster the blood is moving the larger the Doppler shift will be.

> *More precisely, the Doppler shift is determined by how quickly the blood is moving towards or away from the probe.*

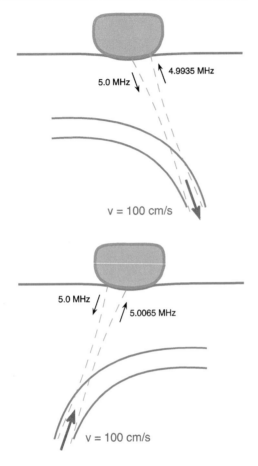

Figure 7.2 Compared with the transmitted frequency, the echoes from blood are slightly lower in frequency if the blood is flowing away from the probe (top), slightly higher in frequency if the blood flow is towards the probe (bottom).

What happens if the direction of movement is not *directly* towards or away from the probe, as shown in Figure 7.3?

In this case we must also take into account the Doppler angle (θ), defined as the angle between the midline of the ultrasound beam and the direction of blood flow.

Thus the Doppler equation, which determines the relationship between the Doppler shift (f_D) and blood velocity (v), is as follows:

$$f_D = \frac{2f(v\cos\theta)}{c}$$

where f is the transmitted ultrasound frequency, c is the propagation speed of ultrasound in soft tissue (1540 m/sec) and θ is the Doppler angle.

The factor of two appears in this equation because the ultrasound travels a round path – from the probe to the blood and from the blood back to the probe – and both of these paths are affected by the movement of the blood.

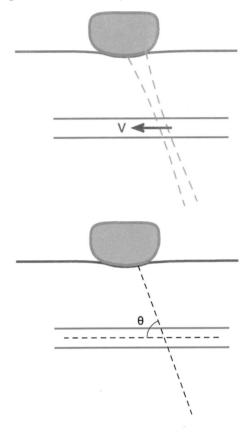

Figure 7.3 Generally flow is at an angle to the beam, not directly towards or away from the probe. It can be shown that the speed of movement towards or away from the probe is given by (v cos θ) where θ is the "Doppler angle".

Looking at the Doppler equation, we can see that some of the parameters in it are known. In particular, the machine knows the frequency it is transmitting (f) and the speed of sound in tissue (c). Thus the Doppler equation can be written as:

$$f_D = \left[\frac{2f}{c}\right] \times (v\cos\theta)$$

where the quantity in square brackets is constant for a given probe frequency and can be calculated by the machine.

Writing the Doppler equation in this way emphasises the fact that the Doppler shift is determined by both the velocity and the direction of blood flow relative to the beam (i.e. the angle θ).

What are typical Doppler shift values? Figure 7.4 shows the Doppler shift for a blood velocity of 100 cm/sec and for a range of probe frequencies and Doppler angles.

Since blood velocities rarely exceed 200 cm/sec, we can see that (by good fortune) the Doppler shift falls within the range of frequencies that can be heard by the human ear. Listening to the Doppler shift has proved to be as useful in Doppler examinations as watching the image is when doing a scan.

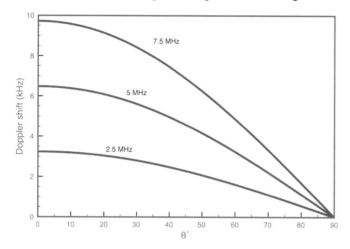

Figure 7.4 The Doppler shift for a blood velocity of 100 cm/sec and for a range of frequencies and Doppler angles. Since cos 90° = 0 there is no Doppler shift when θ = 90°.

The Doppler angle

The importance of the Doppler angle is again highlighted in Figure 7.5.

The basis of Doppler ultrasound is the machine's ability to detect and measure the *Doppler shift*. We usually want it to display *blood velocity*, so the fact that the Doppler shift also depends on the Doppler angle is a problem. How is it dealt with?

There are three possibilities:

(a) measure the Doppler angle and take it into account in the calculation of the blood velocity;

(b) assume the Doppler angle is 0° (i.e. that the beam is aligned with the direction of flow);

(c) the Doppler angle cannot be determined.

We will discuss each of these in turn.

Fortunately in many clinical situations it is possible to determine the Doppler angle reasonably accurately from the grey scale image. Figure 7.6 shows how the user applies "angle correction" to determine the Doppler angle when using spectral pulsed Doppler.

First the Doppler "sample volume" (the region from which Doppler signals will be obtained) is placed in the area of interest. The user then adjusts an "angle marker" to tell the machine the direction of flow.

Since the machine knows the direction of the Doppler beam, it can calculate the Doppler angle (the angle between the direction of the beam and the direction of flow).

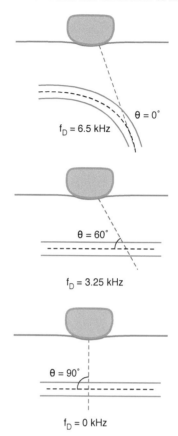

Figure 7.5 Diagram showing the effect of angle on the Doppler shift (as before, probe frequency is 5 MHz and blood velocity is 100 cm/sec).

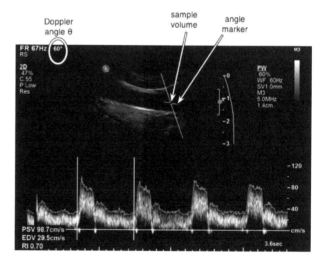

Figure 7.6 Example of a Doppler assessment. The user has placed the sample volume in the centre of the vessel and then aligned the angle marker (the line in the centre of the sample volume) parallel to the vessel walls to indicate the direction of flow. The angle displayed at the top of the screen is 60°.

Now the Doppler equation can be written as:

$$f_D = \left[\frac{2f\cos\theta}{c}\right] \times v$$

The quantity in the square brackets is constant for a given probe frequency and sample volume position and can be calculated by the machine. Rearranging this equation:

$$v = \left[\frac{c}{2f\cos\theta}\right] \times f_D$$

Thus, once the value of the Doppler angle is known the machine can calculate the blood velocity from the measured Doppler shift.

The vertical axis of the spectral display in the lower portion of Figure 7.6 is therefore calibrated in cm/sec, and readings made from this display will also be measured in cm/sec.

In echocardiography the Doppler beam is generally almost parallel to the direction of flow and the machine therefore assumes that the Doppler angle is 0°. In this case the cos θ factor can be ignored since cos 0° = 1.

Indeed for spectral Doppler if the user does not apply angle correction the machine will assume that the Doppler angle is 0° and calculate blood velocity based on this assumption, as shown in Figure 7.7. This can be a trap, since the velocity values will be meaningless if the angle is not 0°.

Sometimes angle correction is not possible.

For example, if we acquire Doppler signals from the small arteries perfusing a region such as the periphery of the kidney, the vessels will generally be too small to be seen in the grey scale image.

What information can we get from the spectral Doppler display in this case?

We still know that the Doppler shift is *proportional* to blood velocity, and thus the variation of the spectral display with time (the "Doppler waveform") accurately represents the time variation of the blood velocity.

A number of indices have been developed to characterise these waveforms and to differentiate between normal and abnormal waveforms. These will be discussed in chapter 9.

We will see later in this chapter that other Doppler modes (colour Doppler and continuous wave Doppler) generally do not lend themselves to angle correction, in which case the effect of Doppler angle remains very important and can be problematic.

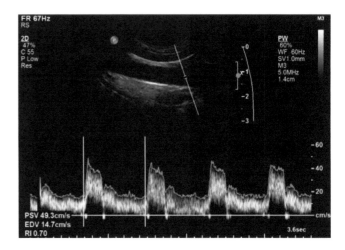

Figure 7.7 (a) If the Doppler has not been angle corrected the velocity scale is calculated assuming that θ = 0°.

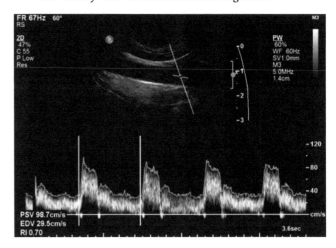

Figure 7.7 (b) After angle correction the scale will read correctly. In this example the angle is 60°. There is a factor of 2 difference between the velocity scales before and after angle correction since cos 60° = 0.5.

Measurement accuracy

Unfortunately the measurement of blood velocity from the Doppler spectral display can never be totally accurate. The main sources of error are:

(a) uncertainty regarding the exact direction of flow;

(b) subjectivity in determining the correct placement of the measurement calipers on the spectral display;

(c) intrinsic spectral broadening, a Doppler artifact which will be discussed later.

The first of these – uncertainty regarding the direction of flow – is particularly important. Careful technique and good equipment design can minimise items (b) and (c).

Why is it not possible to determine the direction of flow accurately?

The dynamics of blood flow are complex (as discussed in chapter 9). One consequence of this complexity is that blood flow is not necessarily parallel to the walls of the blood vessel.

Nevertheless, in normal clinical practice the user places the angle marker parallel with the vessel walls as a "best guess" regarding the direction of flow. As a consequence, it is quite likely that the measured Doppler angle may be incorrect by as much as 5°. What effect does this have on the accuracy of the blood velocity measurement? The answer is that it depends on the value of the Doppler angle being used in the examination. Consider Figure 7.8.

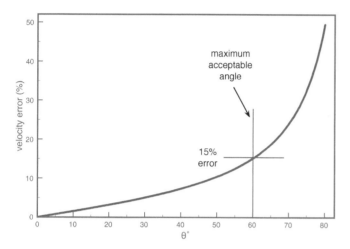

Figure 7.8 Graph indicating the percentage error that would occur in the velocity measurement if there was an angle error of 5°. The error varies dramatically depending on the Doppler angle.

Figure 7.8 shows that the error in velocity is negligible if the Doppler angle is close to 0° (which is fortunate for echocardiographers), but it increases dramatically as the Doppler angle is increased. For this reason:

> *60° is usually considered to be the largest "acceptable" Doppler angle for velocity measurement.*

When the angle is 60° a 5° error in determining the Doppler angle will cause a 15% error in the blood velocity.

Unfortunately in applications other than echocardiography it is not usually possible to achieve an angle close to 0°. Angles close to 60° are more common, so it is important to make measurements with care and to follow protocols closely.

Scattering of ultrasound by blood

Compared to soft tissue, blood is a weak scatterer of ultrasound as shown by the fact that it is normally echo-free in ultrasound images. The only components within the blood that significantly scatter ultrasound are the red cells.

There are two situations where blood becomes more reflective:

(a) when it is stationary or moving very slowly the red cells can clump together in large clusters called "rouleaux"; these reflect ultrasound more strongly than when the red cells are randomly distributed in the blood;

(b) when very small gas bubbles have been intentionally introduced into the blood in the form of an ultrasound contrast agent (this will be discussed in chapter 12).

In general, however, the echoes from blood are very much lower in amplitude than those from tissues. What are the consequences of this poor scattering of blood?

First, to obtain adequate echoes from the blood (and hence adequate Doppler information), the power of the transmitted ultrasound must be higher than in grey scale imaging. This is generally achieved by using a longer transmit pulse duration than is used in imaging. While this degrades the spatial resolution (we saw in an earlier chapter that the shorter the pulse the better the resolution) it has the advantage that it increases the transmitted power without increasing the peak pressure (which could be potentially harmful to the patient's tissues).

Another factor must be taken into account when we consider the exposure of the patient's tissues to ultrasound.

Both pulsed and continuous wave Doppler use a single line of sight, and the ultrasound beam is kept stationary for the duration of the Doppler acquisition. This means that all the transmitted ultrasound energy travels along a single beam and it is therefore concentrated in a small volume of tissue, whereas in grey scale and colour Doppler imaging the beam is scanned and so the energy is spread more widely through the tissues.

This issue will be discussed further in chapter 11.

> *The combination of the increased transmit power and the stationary beam means that the exposure of the patient's tissues to ultrasound is usually higher for pulsed Doppler than for any other mode of operation. Pulsed Doppler is therefore the mode for which the user must be most vigilant regarding safe levels of exposure.*

The poor scattering of ultrasound by blood has another consequence. The tissues adjacent to flowing blood (e.g. blood vessel walls and heart walls) are almost invariably moving as well, due to the dynamics of the blood flow, respiration and (sometimes) probe movement.

Clearly the Doppler-shifted echoes coming from these moving tissues will have much greater amplitude than those from the blood. The Doppler processing must therefore suppress these signals or they would overwhelm the weak blood signals and make them undetectable.

The suppression of Doppler-shifted signals from moving tissue is based on the observation that the speed of movement of the tissues is almost always slower than the blood flow velocity, and hence the Doppler shift of echoes from moving tissues is lower in frequency than that from moving blood.

Doppler signal processing therefore includes a "wall filter" which blocks Doppler signals with frequencies lower than a set cutoff value. The cutoff will vary depending on the application, being lower for venous examinations because vein walls move more slowly than arterial walls. The machine selects a suitable setting for the wall filter cutoff based on the application preset selected, and the user can then change it if necessary during the examination.

Acquisition	Display	Terminology	Group
continuous wave	spectral	continuous wave Doppler CW Doppler	spectral Doppler
pulsed	spectral	pulsed Doppler PW Doppler range-gated Doppler duplex Doppler	spectral Doppler
pulsed	2D colour	colour Doppler	colour Doppler

Table 7.1 The terminology used for Doppler instruments varies considerably.

Suggested activities

1. As you scan take note of some of the vessels you may need to obtain Doppler signals from (e.g. femoral artery, brachial artery, carotid artery, renal artery, aorta, femoral vein, portal vein). Consider whether you could achieve a Doppler angle of 60° or less.

2. Use the Doppler equation to calculate the Doppler shift when a 4 MHz Doppler system is used to detect blood flowing at 50 cm/sec with a Doppler angle of 60°.

3. Suppose the determination of the angle was incorrect, and the true Doppler angle is 57°. Recalculate the Doppler shift and compare the result with the one you calculated above. Calculate the percentage difference caused by this 3° error.

Continuous wave (CW) Doppler

Continuous wave Doppler (generally shortened to "CW Doppler") is the simplest type of Doppler instrument.

Hand-held CW Dopplers can be used stand-alone to detect blood flow in superficial vessels and as fetal heart detectors.

Echocardiographers also use CW Doppler (which is built in to their imaging machine) in cardiac examinations because it can display and measure blood flow velocities in all situations, even when the flow velocity is very high.

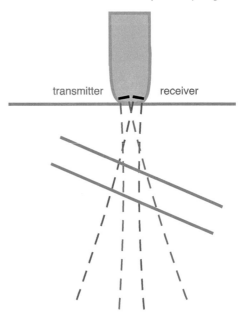

Figure 7.9(a) A typical probe used for hand-held CW Doppler examinations.

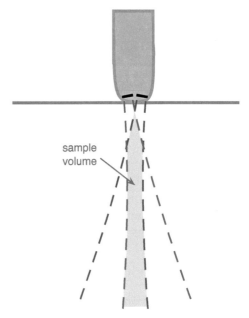

Figure 7.9 (b) The sample volume is defined by the overlap of the transmit and receive beams.

We will see in a later section that while pulsed and colour Doppler have a number of advantages relative to CW Doppler, both are inherently limited in their ability to handle high velocities.

Figure 7.9 shows the principle on which CW Doppler is based. Two separate transducer elements (or groups of elements) are used, one transmitting ultrasound and the other receiving the returning echoes.

This separation of function is needed because (as the name implies) ultrasound is transmitted continuously in CW Doppler, not in pulses as with other modes of operation.

As the diagram shows, the region where the transmit beam and receive beam intersect is termed the "sample volume". Only tissues and blood within this region can produce Doppler shifted echoes that will be detected by the machine, since these are the only tissues that are both exposed to the transmitted ultrasound and "seen" by the receiving transducer.

In general the CW Doppler sample volume is quite large, and it may extend without limit into the tissues. In this case the depth of penetration is limited by attenuation, just as it is for grey scale imaging.

A typical CW Doppler instrument is shown in Figure 7.10.

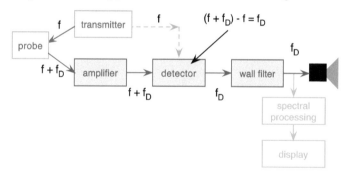

Figure 7.10 Block diagram of a typical CW Doppler. See the text for details.

The transmitter generates a continuous stream of transmitted ultrasound. It also provides a reference signal to the detector so that the transmitted frequency (f) and the frequency of the received echoes ($f + f_D$) can be compared. The detector is the key component – it detects the difference in frequency between its two input signals (the received echo signal and the reference signal from the transmitter), and its output is a signal at the difference frequency $(f + f_D) - f = f_D$ (i.e. the Doppler shift).

Thus the instrument achieves what is needed – it discards the transmitted ultrasound frequency and preserves the Doppler shift in the form of an audible Doppler signal.

After wall filtering (where the part of the signal with frequency below the filter cutoff is removed) the Doppler signal is ready for monitoring and/or display.

Generally it is monitored using a loudspeaker, as shown in the diagram.

Additionally, if the Doppler is built into an imaging machine (as it is in echocardiography) then the signal will be processed to generate a Doppler spectral display similar to the pulsed Doppler spectral displays shown in Figures 7.6 and 7.7.

An extra detail – the direction of flow relative to the probe – must be added to this account. As can be seen in Figure 7.11, the Doppler signal can be displayed above and/or below the zero flow baseline. Conventionally signals are displayed above the line when the direction of flow is towards the probe and below the line when the flow is away from the probe.

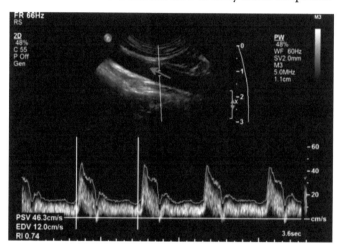

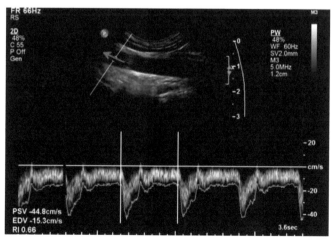

Figure 7.11 The blood in this common carotid artery is flowing from right to left in the image (arrow). (Top) When a pulsed Doppler beam is placed so that flow is towards the probe the spectral display is above the baseline. (Bottom) Conversely, when flow is away from the probe the display is below the baseline.

A technique termed "quadrature detection" is used by the machine to achieve this directional separation. The details of this technique are beyond the scope of this book and will not be discussed further.

The practical question of just how the direction of flow can be determined from the Doppler display is discussed in the next section.

In summary, then, continuous wave Doppler is simple – much simpler than pulsed and colour Doppler, as we will see. It can be very compact and it is often used in the form of a hand-held device such as a fetal heart detector.

In hand-held applications of CW Doppler there is generally no imaging guidance and the device is used "blind". The user's knowledge of anatomy allows the probe to be placed in approximately the right position and then the Doppler signal is the guide to more accurate positioning. In this situation, the relatively large sample volume is an advantage since it means that the positioning does not need to be very precise.

It may be thought that the transmitted power of CW Doppler would be very high, as the ultrasound is transmitted continuously, but this is not the case because the amplitude is reduced to compensate for this fact.

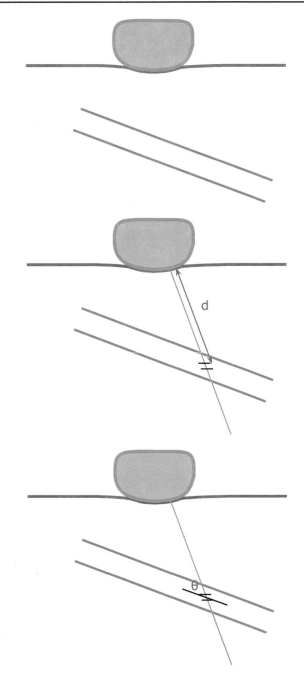

Pulsed Doppler

The main limitation of CW Doppler is its inability to accurately define the sample volume (the volume of tissue from which the Doppler signals come).

Pulsed Doppler (sometimes called "pulse wave" or "range gated" Doppler) was developed to address this shortcoming.

Pulsed Doppler can accurately define the location of a small sample volume having dimensions of typically a few millimetres. Moreover, since it is used in combination with grey scale imaging, the sample volume can be positioned by the user anywhere within the grey scale image, as Figures 7.6, 7.7, 7.11 and 7.12 demonstrate.

Yet another advantage of pulsed Doppler is that it is possible to angle correct, as shown in Figure 7.7 and 7.12, except when the direction of flow is unknown.

As discussed earlier, angle correction allows the machine to determine the Doppler angle θ; as long as θ is less than 60° and the angle has been accurately measured, valid readings of blood velocity can then be obtained from the Doppler spectral display.

Figure 7.12 (Top) The vessel of interest is identified in the grey scale image. (Centre) The user places the sample volume within the vessel. This allows the machine to calculate the necessary beam direction and sample volume depth (d) that it must use. (Bottom) The user then positions the angle marker parallel to the vessel walls, enabling the machine to calculate the Doppler angle (θ).

Pulsed Doppler relies on the "pulse echo principle", the same principle that is the basis of grey scale imaging. This refers to the machine's ability to relate the arrival time of an echo to the depth of the structure causing the echo. Since this principle is used in both pulsed Doppler and grey scale imaging it is not surprising that they can be used in combination so effectively.

As Figure 7.12 shows, once the user has positioned the sample volume the machine can determine the beam direction and sample volume depth needed. If angle correction has been applied then the machine will also determine the Doppler angle.

Pulsed Doppler data acquisition can then begin.

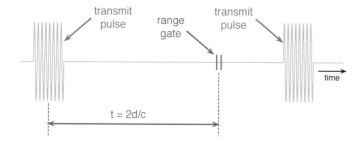

Figure 7.13 (a) The machine waits a fixed time after each transmit pulse and then samples the echo signals briefly using a "range gate". The time delay (t) between the transmit pulse and the range gate is calculated to ensure that the echoes come from the correct depth.

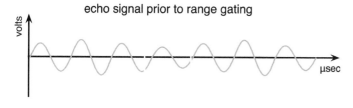

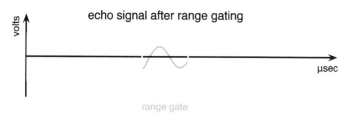

Figure 7.13 (b) Both the time scale and the amplitude have been magnified to show more detail of the range gating process. The only part of the echo signal retained for further processing is the short interval within the time span of the range gate. Echoes from tissues nearer to the probe than the range gate and deeper than it are ignored.

After each transmit pulse (see Figure 7.13) the machine waits a fixed amount of time (*t*) and then briefly acquires a short "sample" of the echo signal (typically one or two microseconds in duration). This process is termed "range gating". The delay time between the transmit pulse and the range gate is calculated by the machine so that the signal comes from the required sample volume depth (*d*).

Echoes which arrive earlier and later than the range gate are completely ignored.

The transmit-receive cycle repeats regularly. This is similar to grey scale imaging except the beam does not move. The range gate captures another sample of the echoes from the depth *d* each time.

The number of transmit-receive cycles each second is the Doppler PRF (pulse repetition frequency).

The echo samples acquired from a number of successive transmit pulses are combined electronically (see Figure 7.14). The result is a Doppler signal essentially identical to that which would be have been obtained if a CW Doppler was able to look selectively at the blood within the sample volume.

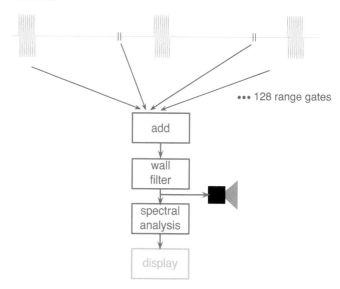

Figure 7.14 Echo samples acquired from a number of successive range gates (typically 128) are combined electronically, creating a Doppler signal. The signal is wall filtered and it can then be monitored and displayed.

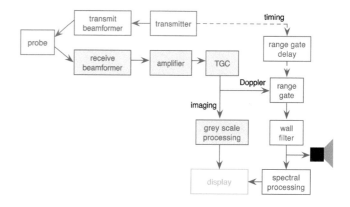

Figure 7.15 Block diagram showing pulsed Doppler incorporated into a grey scale imaging machine. Note the timing information required to inform the Doppler system when the transmit pulse has been sent so it can calculate the range gate timing correctly.

The pulsed Doppler signal is wall filtered, monitored by loudspeaker and processed to produce a spectral display, just as is done with the CW Doppler signal in echocardiography.

Figure 7.15 shows in block diagram form how pulsed Doppler is incorporated into a grey scale imaging machine.

In summary, pulsed Doppler allows a small range gate to be placed accurately in an area of interest, and it then provides detailed Doppler shift information regarding the dynamics of flow within that sample volume. Its major disadvantages are that the exposure of the patient to ultrasound is higher than in other ultrasound modalities and it is limited in its ability to detect very high velocities (this will be discussed shortly).

Spectral display

Why is the spectral display so widely used for Doppler signals? To answer this we need to understand the nature of the Doppler signal and how it is affected by the detailed dynamics of blood flow.

Consider a pulsed Doppler sample volume placed within a blood vessel, as shown in Figure 7.16. The sample volume size is determined by the beamwidth, the transmit pulse duration and the range gate duration. Typically this volume contains millions of moving red cells at any instant, each contributing to the Doppler shifted echo received by the machine.

Most importantly, these red cells will not all be moving at the same velocity. Instead, blood velocity will vary across the vessel, generally being highest at the centre and reducing to very low velocities near the walls (as shown in Figure 7.16). (This "velocity profile" will be discussed in chapter 9.)

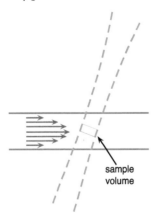

Figure 7.16 The pulsed Doppler sample volume can occupy a significant fraction of the area of the blood vessel, and hence it "sees" a range of blood velocities (arrows).

The Doppler signal will therefore contain a range of Doppler shift frequencies reflecting the range of red cell velocities within the sample volume.

The main advantage of the spectral display is that it shows the detailed distribution of frequencies in the Doppler signal and how the signal changes with time.

We will see in chapter 9 that in the presence of disease it is common for both the blood velocity and the distribution of velocities to change. These changes will alter the Doppler signal in ways that can be clearly recognised and quantified in the spectral display.

Figure 7.17 shows the spectral display in its most basic form where the vertical axis (Doppler shift) is calibrated in frequency units and the display range is distributed equally above and below the baseline.

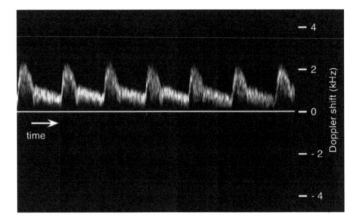

Figure 7.17 A Doppler spectral display where the vertical axis is calibrated in frequency units. (PRF = 8 kHz, f = 5 MHz, θ = 60°)

As discussed above, the convention is that when the signals are displayed above the baseline this means that flow is towards the probe while signals below the line mean that flow is away from the probe. A minus sign on the axis markings also indicates flow away from the probe.

Note that the user can invert the display for convenience, in which case flow towards the probe is below the baseline and flow away from the probe is above the line. This may be done, for example, when viewing an arterial signal where flow is away from the probe.

It is important to recognise that the direction of flow can change in disease. For example, the direction of flow in the main portal vein may reverse in patients with portal hypertension. It is therefore essential that the user can correctly determine the direction of blood flow from the Doppler display.

How is this done?

Consider the common carotid artery Doppler signal shown in Figure 7.18. It is often easiest to proceed as follows:

(i) Decide what is the expected direction of flow in the vessel.

(ii) Taking into account the Doppler beam orientation, determine whether flow in this direction would be seen by the machine as being towards or away from the probe (see Figures 7.18 (b) and 7.19).

(iii) Now look at the Doppler trace to see whether the machine is displaying flow towards or away from the probe. Is it consistent with the assumed direction of flow in the vessel? If yes then you have confirmed the assumed direction of flow; if not then flow must be in the opposite direction.

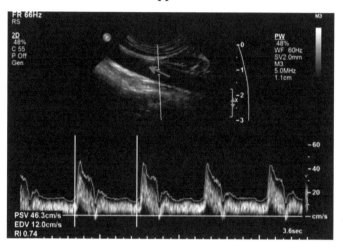

Figure 7.18 (a) A Doppler signal acquired from the common carotid artery. The spectrum is displayed above the baseline, and the numbers on the vertical axis are positive (there is no minus sign), confirming that the blood is flowing towards the probe.

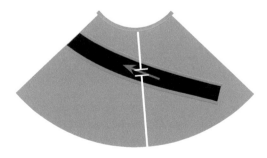

Figure 7.18 (b) The expected direction of flow in this artery is from right to left (i.e. from the heart to the head). For the Doppler beam direction shown the blood will be seen by the machine as flowing towards the probe.

As an example, let us apply this methodology to the common carotid artery in Figure 7.18.

(i) The blood should be flowing from right to left (see Figure 7.18 (b)).

(ii) Flow in this direction would be displayed as flow towards the probe.

(iii) This is what we see in the display, so our assumption about the direction of flow has been confirmed – it is going from right to left.

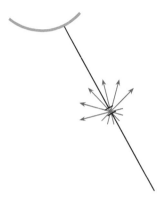

Figure 7.19 (a) Blood flow in any of the directions shown by the red arrows will be seen as flow towards the probe.

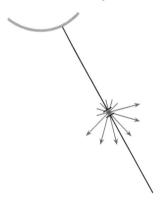

Figure 7.19 (b) Flow in any of these directions will be seen as flow away from the probe.

The upper and lower limits of the spectral display are particularly important. These determine the maximum possible Doppler shifts that can be correctly measured and displayed. They are called the "Nyquist Limits" and their value is equal to one half of the Doppler PRF.

Clearly increasing or decreasing the PRF (i.e. the number of Doppler transmit pulses per second) will increase or decrease the range of frequencies that can be displayed. A standard user control in pulsed Doppler (and colour Doppler) is therefore the "velocity scale". This control simply increases or decreases the Doppler PRF thus altering the range of Doppler shift frequencies that can be displayed.

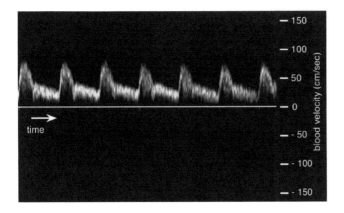

Figure 7.20 The spectral display shown in Figure 7.17 has now been angle corrected, and so the vertical axis is marked in velocity units (cm/sec).

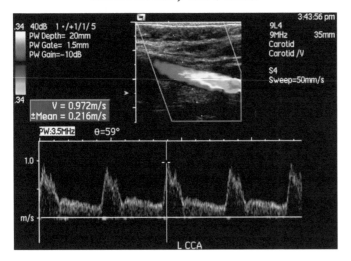

Figure 7.21 (a) Measurements can be made manually by positioning a measurement marker on the upper edge of the spectral display.

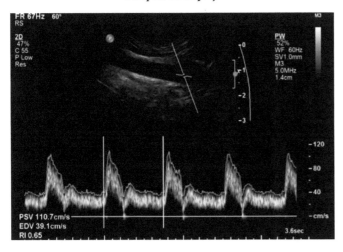

Figure 7.21 (b) Some machines can make measurements automatically. Here the envelope of the spectrum has been traced by the machine and a single heart cycle identified. This has enabled the machine to measure the peak systolic velocity (PSV) and end diastolic velocity (EDV) and to calculate an index from them (the Resistance Index RI).

Other pulsed Doppler controls include the sample volume length (which varies the duration of the range gate), Doppler gain and wall filter cutoff frequency.

As mentioned above, the user will apply angle correction whenever possible so that the velocity of blood flow can be determined. The vertical scale of the spectral display will then be calibrated in blood velocity units (as shown in Figure 7.20) rather than frequency units (as shown in Figure 7.17).

As Figure 7.21 shows, measurements are made from the upper edge or "envelope" of the spectral display. For arterial signals, typical measured values are the peak systolic velocity and the minimum and/or end diastolic velocity.

Suggested activities

1. Experiment with the following Doppler controls, noting their effect on the audible signal and the spectral display: Doppler gain (find what setting of this control gives the cleanest Doppler signal); wall filter cutoff; velocity scale; sweep speed (time scale); sample volume length.

2. Rotate the angle marker slightly to alter the measured Doppler angle by a few degrees and note the effect on the spectral display's velocity scale.

3. Freeze a spectral trace and make repeated measurements of the peak velocity to see how reproducible your measurements are.

Colour Doppler

CW and pulsed Doppler provide detailed information about the blood flow within a single sample volume.

Colour Doppler does something very different. It creates a real-time two-dimensional image where Doppler shift information is coded in colour and overlaid on the grey scale image. Figure 7.22 shows a typical example.

> *It is important to remember that the colour represents Doppler shift, not blood flow velocity. Thus the colour displayed at each point depends on both the blood velocity and the Doppler angle at that point.*

We will return to this issue later.

To create this two-dimensional Doppler image the machine must rapidly measure the Doppler shift at a large number of points within the colour box. The Doppler shift determines the colour that will be displayed at each point.

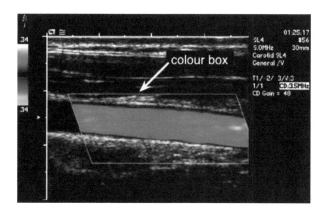

Figure 7.22 A colour Doppler image. Colour is displayed only within the colour box and only where flowing blood is found. Standard grey scale information is displayed everywhere else. The sides of the colour box are angled, indicating that the beam has been steered during Doppler acquisition to ensure a suitable Doppler angle.

To start a colour Doppler examination the user adjusts the position and size of the colour box so that it encompasses the region of interest. The Doppler controls are checked and colour Doppler imaging can begin.

The machine starts by creating a grey scale image in the normal way (see Figure 7.23).

It then acquires the colour image by scanning the ultrasound beam through the tissues within the colour box, collecting Doppler shift information at each point. The Doppler information is overlaid on the grey scale image to produce the colour Doppler image.

The machine alternates rapidly between grey scale and colour image acquisition so that many colour Doppler images can be created each second.

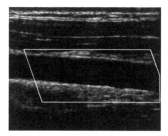 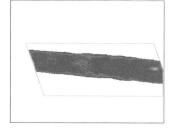

Figure 7.23 The machine starts with a grey scale image (left). It then acquires colour information for the tissues within the colour box (right). The two images are combined to create the colour Doppler image in Figure 7.22.

How is the Doppler information acquired? As Figure 7.24 shows, a large number of sample volumes are created along each beam, spanning from top to bottom of the colour box. This allows the machine to determine the Doppler shift in all of these sample volumes at the same time.

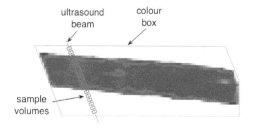

Figure 7.24 An expanded view of the colour image showing that it is composed of blocks of colour, each determined by the Doppler shift detected in one of the colour Doppler sample volumes.

Colour Doppler is based on the same range gating principle as spectral pulsed Doppler, but differs from it in several ways:

1. Only a small number of transmit pulses (e.g. 8) are used to acquire the Doppler information for each line of sight (beam position). This is very different from pulsed Doppler which typically uses 128 pulses for each determination of the Doppler shift.

2. A large number of range gates operate, each with a different time delay (see Figures 7.24 and 7.25).

3. The processing of the echo information for each range gate is quite different from that used in pulsed Doppler (see Figures 7.25 and 7.26). A calculation is made using the 8 echo samples. The result of this calculation is just three numbers which are measures of (i) the mean Doppler shift frequency, (ii) the "variance" and (iii) the Doppler signal power. The use of these parameters will be discussed shortly.

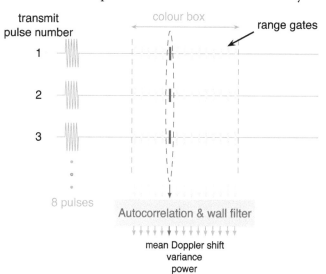

Figure 7.25 For a given beam position a total of 8 transmit pulses are used. A series of range gates corresponding to the sample volumes in Figure 7.24 are used to sample the echo information for each transmit pulse. The 8 echo samples for each range gate are processed to yield the three colour Doppler parameters shown.

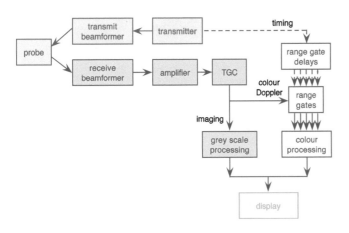

Figure 7.26 Block diagram showing colour Doppler processing incorporated into a grey scale imaging machine.

Note that there is no Doppler signal as such, and hence there is there is no audible output or spectral display.

We saw above that speed is essential for colour Doppler, both in acquiring the echo data and in processing and displaying it. Fast acquisition of the echo data is achieved by:

- using a small number of pulses (e.g. 8) for each line of sight,
- collecting echo information from many range gates at the same time,
- restricting the colour information to the colour box and
- making the colour box relatively narrow.

As discussed above, fast processing and display is achieved by calculating just three parameters for each sample volume. What do these three parameters mean and how are they used by the machine to determine what is displayed?

The mean (or average) Doppler shift is the most important as it determines the colour displayed at each point in the colour image. It is *proportional* to the mean blood velocity within the sample volume but it also depends on the Doppler angle at that point.

By convention, red colours are used when flow is towards the probe and blue when flow is away from the probe. As the colour bar on the machine's display shows (see Figure 7.27), the colour varies to indicate the amount of Doppler shift, ranging from dark shades of red and blue for low velocities to lighter shades for high velocities. Areas where flow is absent or too slow to be detected are black.

The range of Doppler shifts that can be measured and displayed is constrained by the Nyquist Limit (half the Doppler PRF), just as it is for spectral pulsed Doppler.

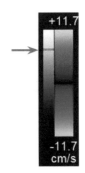

Figure 7.27 The colour bar shows the range of colours used to display the various Doppler shifts. Colours above the baseline correspond to flow towards the probe, as in the spectral display. Note also the grey scale bar to the left of the colour bar (arrow); this is related to the tissue/blood discrimination function.

Note that the velocity values displayed at the top and bottom of the colour bar indicate what the blood velocity *would be* at the Nyquist limits *if the Doppler angle was 0°*. It is important to recognise that these values are incorrect and of no real use if the Doppler angle is not 0°.

The second parameter, the "variance" of the Doppler signal, is a measure of spectral broadening. In most colour Doppler applications it is not displayed, although it is used in the tissue/blood discrimination function as discussed shortly. In echocardiography, on the other hand, areas of unusually large variance (i.e. areas with increased spectral broadening) are highlighted in the display using an additional colour, usually green (see Figure 7.28).

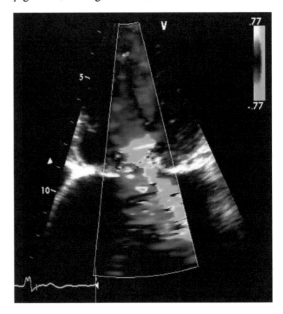

Figure 7.28 A colour Doppler image of the heart showing the use of variance (displayed in green) to highlight areas with increased spectral broadening. This is likely to be caused by turbulence.

The third parameter is the Doppler signal power. This is simply a measure of how strong the Doppler signal from each sample volume is. Like the variance, it is used in the tissue/blood discrimination function. In addition, the power is the parameter that is colour-coded and displayed in a specialised version of colour Doppler known as "power mode" colour Doppler. This will be discussed shortly.

Figure 7.29 is a block diagram showing the colour Doppler processing in more detail.

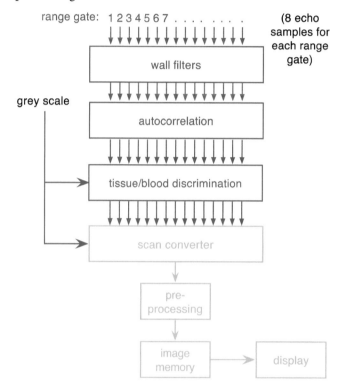

Figure 7.29 Block diagram showing in more detail the colour Doppler processing and image formation.

With reference to Figure 7.29, let us walk through the colour processing for a single range gate.

The 8 echo samples from the range gate are first wall-filtered to remove, as far as possible, any Doppler signals caused by moving tissues.

Unfortunately the colour Doppler wall filter is less effective than the pulsed Doppler wall filter because it has far less data to work with (just 8 samples). Thus Doppler signals from moving tissues will not be completely eliminated, and they will need to be suppressed later in the processing (specifically by the tissue/blood discrimination function).

Following the wall filter, the echoes are processed using the autocorrelation function to yield the three Doppler parameters discussed earlier – the mean Doppler shift, variance and power.

As with spectral Doppler, quadrature processing is used to determine whether flow is towards or away from the probe.

In the tissue/blood discrimination processor the machine analyses these three Doppler parameters, together with the grey scale echo amplitude at the same point, to determine whether the display should show grey scale (i.e. tissue) or colour (blood flow) at that point.

If the machine determines that the range gate has sampled moving blood and produced valid Doppler information then the mean Doppler shift will be displayed. If it does not, then the grey scale echo will be displayed in the normal way and the colour information for that point will be ignored.

How does the tissue/blood discrimination function work? First the machine assesses the strength of the grey scale echo. If it is stronger than a preset threshold value then the decision is made that tissue is present at that point in the image and so the grey scale information is displayed.

The threshold value for this "grey scale priority" (or "tissue priority") function is preset by the machine, but it can be adjusted by the user. Its value is displayed as a horizontal line on the grey scale bar located next to the colour bar, as shown in Figure 7.27. If the grey scale threshold is increased then stronger grey scale echoes will be required to override the display of colour. If it is decreased then lower level grey scale echoes will override the colour. If the grey scale echo is below the threshold value then the tissue/blood decision is based on the three measured Doppler parameters instead.

Before the colour image is stored in the memory the preprocessor fills any gaps and smooths the image. Persistence may also be used to improve the appearance of the colour image.

In summary, colour Doppler is a valuable and widely used modality. Its obvious strength is the two-dimensional display of Doppler information.

Its applications include:

- locating vessels;
- guiding the placement of the sample volume for a pulsed Doppler examination;
- identifying interconnections between vessels;
- mapping the relationship of vessels to organs;
- assessing the vascularity of a region (e.g. around a suspected malignancy);
- highlighting areas where the blood flow is potentially abnormal.

Colour Doppler also plays a major role in echocardiography.

However, we have seen that colour Doppler has a number of limitations, many of them related to the need to collect and process the echo data quickly for each colour image. The use of a small number of transmit pulses for each colour line of sight (e.g. 8) limits colour Doppler in a number of ways.

Compared with spectral pulsed Doppler, colour Doppler:

- is less able to detect slow-moving blood (so the velocity scale must be optimised at all times);
- is less successful in removing signals caused by moving tissues;
- measures the Doppler shift less accurately.

When the region of interest is relatively deep the colour Doppler frame rate may be quite low. This is clearly a disadvantage in a modality which we often use to assess highly dynamic cardiac and arterial blood flow. What can be done to improve the frame rate?

Generally the machine is designed to use a coarser "line density" (i.e. distance between lines of sight) when acquiring colour Doppler than for grey scale imaging. Some machines even offer the user a control allowing priority to be placed on either spatial resolution (finer line density) or frame rate (coarser line density).

Some machines have the capability to form several beams simultaneously, as discussed in chapter 12. If, for example, four beams are formed this will increase the frame rate by a factor of four.

Another parameter is the width of the colour box. The narrower it is the less lines of sight will be needed to create each image and so the frame rate will be higher.

What about the exposure of the patient's tissues to ultrasound? Colour Doppler exposures are generally somewhat higher than for grey scale imaging due to the increased transmit power needed to get adequate echoes from the blood. However, the exposure will be lower than for pulsed Doppler since the beam sweeps through a volume of tissue while in pulsed Doppler it is stationary. Note that when the colour box is made very narrow the exposure will be increased since it is concentrated in a smaller volume of tissue.

There are two further limitations of colour Doppler. First, it should be clear that colour Doppler is relatively complex and must be optimised for each examination.

While the machine's presets are often adequate, fine tuning of the controls is essential, especially in demanding situations (e.g. where the question is whether or not there is a trickle of blood flow through an occluded or nearly-occluded vessel.)

Secondly, the Doppler angle will usually vary throughout the image, making it virtually impossible to interpret the colours displayed except in a qualitative way. Figure 7.30 shows a dramatic example.

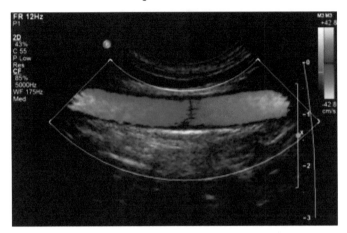

Figure 7.30 The colours vary continuously along the length of this straight vessel. The blood velocity is the same throughout; the changing colour is entirely due to the changing Doppler angle.

The inability to angle correct at each point and the other limitations of colour Doppler discussed above mean that as a modality it is complementary to spectral pulsed Doppler, not a substitute for it. When detailed information is needed (e.g. in an area identified on colour Doppler as being suspicious) pulsed Doppler must be used.

Power mode colour Doppler

The colour Doppler display can be complex and confusing at times due to the colour variations caused by changes in Doppler shift and flow direction (see Figures 7.30 and 7.31).

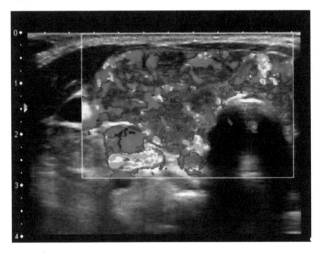

Figure 7.31 A colour Doppler image showing thyroid vascularity. Note how the variations in colour make it difficult to get an overall feel for the distribution and density of the vessels.

In some situations displaying the Doppler shift does not add value, in which case a simpler form of colour Doppler, "power mode" colour Doppler, can be more effective. Figure 7.32 shows two examples.

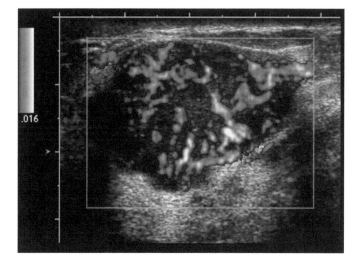

Figure 7.32 (a) A power mode colour Doppler image showing the vascularity in a breast mass. Compared to Figure 7.31 it is much easier to assess the distribution of the vessels in this image. Note the colour bar now shows how the colour varies with signal strength.

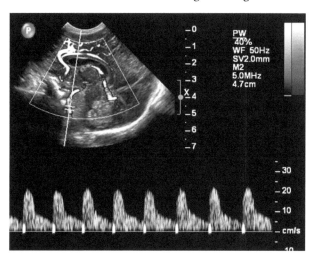

Figure 7.32 (b) Here a power mode colour Doppler image has been used to guide the placement of a pulsed Doppler sample volume in a neonatal brain.

How is the power mode colour Doppler image made? The processing is identical to that used for standard colour Doppler except that the colour displayed is determined by the Doppler signal power (i.e. how strong it is) rather than the mean Doppler shift.

In some machines it is possible to retain information about whether the flow is towards or away from the probe and so a directional power mode image can be displayed, as shown in Figure 7.33.

By good fortune, power mode colour Doppler has other advantages:

- Power mode colour Doppler is significantly more sensitive than standard colour Doppler, so it is the preferred mode when weak signals need to be detected and displayed. The reason for this is that it is easier for the machine to reliably determine the signal power than the mean Doppler shift when the echo signal is weak.

- With power mode colour Doppler, flow is detected and displayed even when the Doppler angle is 90° and there is no real Doppler shift. This is due to the presence of an artifact, "spectral mirror artifact", which will be discussed in chapter 8. Note that the flow would *not* be detected with conventional colour Doppler since the mean Doppler shift in this situation is zero.

- It is not affected by aliasing, except when the directional display is used.

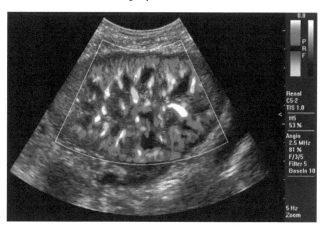

Figure 7.33 Directional power mode colour Doppler image showing the distribution of blood vessels in a transplant kidney.

Thus power mode colour Doppler is a specialised form of colour Doppler used in specific settings. Its advantages are that the display is simpler, the colour image does not drop out when the Doppler angle is 90° and it is possible to detect weak signals more reliably.

Doppler Tissue Imaging

Doppler Tissue Imaging (or DTI) is another specialised application of colour Doppler. The processing is identical to standard colour Doppler except that the wall filtering is reversed.

Doppler signals from moving tissue are retained and signals from moving blood are suppressed. The result is a colour coded image of moving tissues, as shown in Figure 7.34.

In addition to colour coding the grey scale image of the heart, DTI can also be used to produce a colour coded M-mode, as Figure 7.34 shows.

Furthermore, it is often reasonable to assume that the Doppler angle is close to 0°, in which case the Doppler shift values can be converted into velocity values.

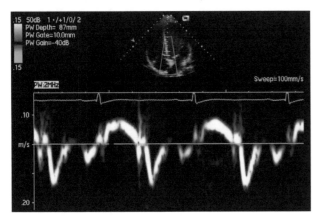

Figure 7.34 An example of Doppler Tissue Imaging. Here it has been used to identify the medial mitral annulus and then to obtain a spectral tracing showing its motion. Its main application is in the assessment of cardiac dynamics.

Suggested activities

1. Experiment with the following colour Doppler controls: velocity scale, gain, tissue priority, wall filter, colour box size (both width and depth). Observe the colour image as you do this and see what settings give the best image.

2. Obtain a colour Doppler image of an artery and optimise it. Without changing the colour settings, move the probe so that a vein is being imaged instead. Observe whether the flow in the vein is well displayed. Re-optimise the image for the vein (e.g. by lowering the velocity scale and wall filter cutoff) and note any improvement in the colour image quality.

3. Compare conventional colour Doppler with power mode colour Doppler in a variety of situations. Note their relative strengths and weaknesses.

Chapter 8

Doppler artifacts

Spectral Doppler artifacts

A number of specific artifacts occur with spectral Doppler ultrasound. The most important is frequency aliasing, which occurs with pulsed Doppler in the presence of high velocities. It also occurs with colour Doppler as we will see later in this chapter.

Frequency aliasing

Abnormally high velocities most commonly occur as a result of arterial and valvular stenosis (narrowing of arteries and heart valves). To diagnose and assess stenosis it is therefore essential that these high velocities be measured.

Clearly the fact that pulsed Doppler is limited in its ability to display and measure high velocities is a serious problem.

We saw in chapter 7 that there is a fixed limit on the range of Doppler shifts that can be correctly displayed. This limit is called the Nyquist Limit and it is equal to one half of the Doppler PRF.

What happens if the Doppler shift exceeds this limit?

The display is "aliased" and the Doppler information appears to suddenly change both its direction and velocity. Fortunately it is very easy to recognise the appearance of aliasing in the spectral display (see Figure 8.1).

When and why does frequency aliasing occur? Broadly speaking, it occurs whenever the pulsed Doppler processor gets insufficient information to correctly determine the Doppler shift. What defines "sufficient"? The machine will correctly detect and display Doppler information *as long as the PRF is at least twice the highest Doppler shift.*

Stating this mathematically, for proper detection and display of the Doppler shift we require:

$$PRF > 2f_D$$

Rearranging this equation, we require:

$$f_D < \frac{PRF}{2}$$

We can recognise (PRF/2) as the Nyquist Limit. When this limit is violated (i.e. when the Doppler shift exceeds the Nyquist Limit) the machine makes an incorrect "guess" about the Doppler frequency, as shown in Figure 8.2 and so aliasing occurs, as shown in Figure 8.3.

You may have noticed that in television scenes wheels often seem to rotate backwards. This is visual aliasing. It occurs because the television frame rate (the number of pictures per second) is too low to correctly capture the true motion of the wheel.

Since aliasing is an important limitation of pulsed Doppler, we need to explore whether there are ways to reduce or eliminate it. Imagine that the spectral display in Figure 8.3 was printed on paper. It would be quite straightforward to cut off the lower portion of the display (ranging from -0.5 kHz downwards) and place it above the upper part of the display, being careful to superimpose the lines representing the Nyquist Limits.

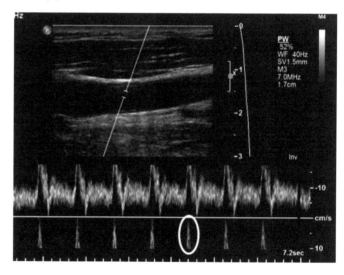

Figure 8.1 An example of a spectral display with aliasing. The peaks of the arterial waveform are cut off and displaced to the bottom of the display (circled).

The result (see Figure 8.4) would be that the display would be altered in such a way that the aliased signal would no longer appear to be aliased.

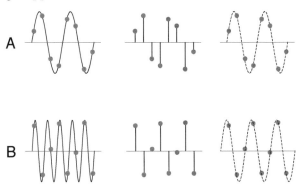

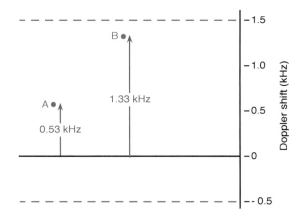

Figure 8.4 Shifting the baseline of the spectral display allows the higher frequency (B) to be displayed correctly. Note that the display range above the baseline has been increased at the cost of a reduced range below the line.

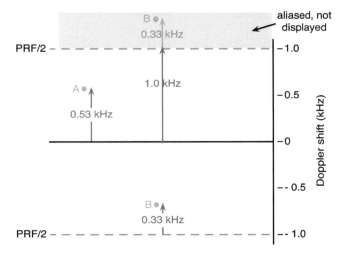

Figure 8.2 The Doppler signal is "sampled" by the range gate at regular intervals (left). The machine takes these sample values (centre) and fits an assumed Doppler signal to them (right). (A) If the Doppler frequency is less than the Nyquist Limit the reconstructed Doppler signal is a perfect replica of the original. (B) If the frequency exceeds the Nyquist Limit, the reconstructed signal has an entirely different frequency to the original.

The machine therefore provides the user with a control allowing the baseline to be moved up or down so that the majority of the spectral display range is in one direction or the other.

When the baseline is shifted the display range in the opposite direction is reduced.

Is this a problem? No. In general the high velocity is directed in just one direction and flow in the opposite direction will be far lower in velocity.

A clinical example of baseline shifting is shown in Figure 8.5.

Figure 8.3 On the spectral display the lower Doppler frequency shift A (0.53 kHz) is correctly displayed, but the higher frequency B (1.33 kHz) has been aliased since it exceeds the Nyquist Limit of 1.0 kHz. It is therefore incorrectly displayed at the bottom of the screen.

Measurement of the previously aliased Doppler shift would now yield the correct Doppler shift or velocity value. (It should be noted that aliasing is still in fact occurring, but its effect is now concealed in the display.)

Thus both the appearance of the display and the numerical value of the Doppler shift can be "corrected" using this simple display trick.

Baseline shifting is therefore the first line of defence when aliasing occurs, or is likely to occur.

Are there limits on baseline shifting? Yes. If the Doppler signal is larger than the PRF (i.e. more than double the Nyquist Limit) then the aliased signal will cross over the baseline as shown in Figure 8.6 and baseline shifting will not be able to eliminate it.

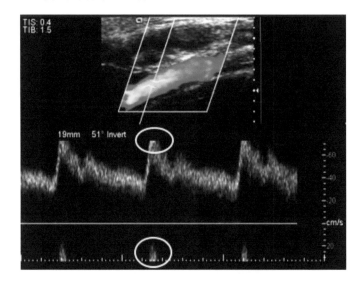

Figure 8.5 (a) Doppler spectral waveform showing aliasing (circled).

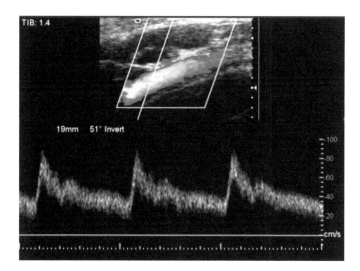

Figure 8.5 (b) The baseline has been shifted down, eliminating the effect of aliasing. Note the baseline has been moved close to the bottom of the display.

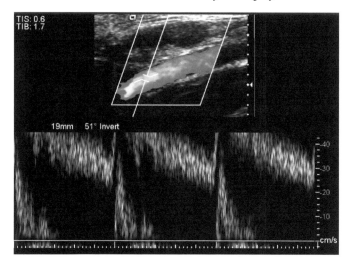

Figure 8.6 Here the maximum Doppler shift is greater than the PRF (i.e. twice the Nyquist Limit), causing severe aliasing that cannot be removed by baseline shifting.

What else can be done to reduce or eliminate aliasing? There are a number of options:

1. Increase the velocity scale (i.e. the Doppler PRF). Remember, however, that the PRF is limited by the depth of penetration, as discussed in chapter 3. The deeper the penetration the lower this limit is. In some machines a "high PRF" mode of operation may be available where the PRF can be increased beyond this limit; this is discussed in more detail below.

2. Find another acoustic window which brings the target vessel closer to the probe so that a higher PRF can be used.

3. Use a lower probe frequency. Since the Doppler

equation states that the Doppler shift generated by a given velocity is directly proportional to the ultrasound frequency, it follows that reducing the probe frequency (e.g. from 4.0 MHz to 3.0 MHz) will reduce the Doppler shift and so it will reduce or eliminate aliasing.

4. Increase the Doppler angle. While this will reduce the Doppler shift it is often not feasible, either because the acoustic window to the vessel is too limited to allow much angle variation or because the angle is close to 60° and so it should not be increased further.

5. In echocardiography CW Doppler is often used instead of pulsed Doppler. Since CW Doppler measures the Doppler shift continuously it is not affected by aliasing. As we have seen, its disadvantage is its relatively large sample volume. However, aliasing occurs when the velocity of interest is very high and so lower Doppler shift signals from elsewhere in the sample volume are unlikely to interfere with the display and measurement of the high velocity signal (as shown in Figure 8.7).

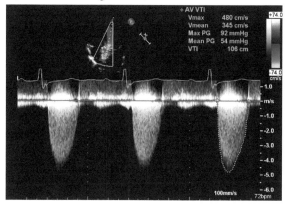

Figure 8.7 An example of the use of CW Doppler in the heart. Here it is being used to measure a high velocity jet caused by aortic stenosis. Although a mixture of signals is displayed, the signal of interest (the very high velocity flow away from the transducer reaching almost 5 m/sec) can easily be seen and measured.

"High PRF" mode and range ambiguity

In pulsed Doppler the PRF is generally limited (just as it is for grey scale imaging) by the requirement that the machine must wait until all detectable echoes have been received before it transmits again (see Figure 8.8 (a)). There is no uncertainty regarding the depth from which each echo comes.

If this rule is violated, an artifact known as "range ambiguity" occurs, since it is no longer clear which transmit pulse gave rise to any given echo.

In grey scale imaging this would lead to duplication of tissue echoes at another depth, which can be very confusing and is considered unacceptable. In pulsed Doppler range ambiguity also occurs, but the consequences are often considered acceptable.

Thus, when other measures have failed to eliminate aliasing, many machines permit the user to increase the Doppler PRF beyond the usual limit. The machine is then said to be operating in "high PRF" mode, and range ambiguity will occur (see Figure 8.8 (b)).

As Figure 8.8 demonstrates, in high PRF mode the Doppler signal will consist of a mixture of signals from the desired sample volume (at depth d_1) and from a second unwanted sample volume (closer to the probe at depth d_2).

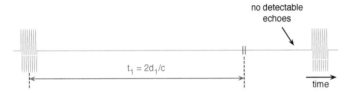

Figure 8.8 (a) Normally the machine waits until all detectable echoes have been received before it transmits again. This ensures that the next transmit pulse cannot occur until after the range gate, so there is no ambiguity regarding the depth d_1 from which the Doppler signal has been acquired.

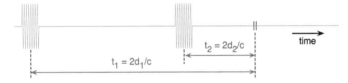

Figure 8.8 (b) In high PRF mode, however, the next transmit pulse can occur during the range gate delay time t_1. Echoes from the desired depth (d_1) will still be sampled correctly by the range gate, however echoes from a shallower depth d_2 will also be detected due to the second transmit pulse.

Generally the ultrasound machine will indicate the second sample volume in the image (as shown in Figure 8.9) to alert the user to its existence.

Would we expect this second range gate to cause problems? Generally no. The argument is identical to that regarding the use of CW Doppler in the heart. If interfering signals are detected in the unwanted sample volume they will almost certainly be much lower in Doppler shift and hence they will not interfere with the display and measurement of the signal of interest.

Figure 8.9 shows a clinical example of high PRF Doppler.

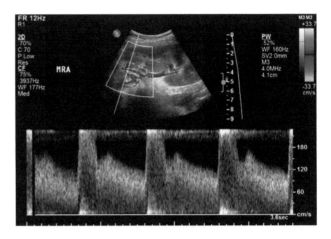

Figure 8.9 (a) This spectral waveform is still severely aliased despite baseline shifting and other measures aimed at removing the aliasing.

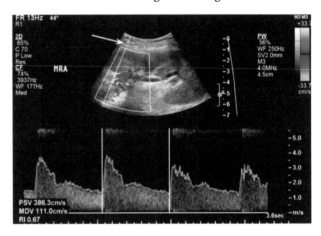

Figure 8.9 (b) High PRF mode eliminates the aliasing, although it introduces an unwanted second sample volume closer to the probe (arrow).

Intrinsic spectral broadening

A less well-known Doppler artifact is intrinsic spectral broadening. An example is shown in Figure 8.10.

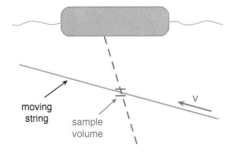

Figure 8.10 (a) In a moving string Doppler phantom the signal comes from a thread moving in water at a controlled speed. In this experiment the velocity of the string was increased and decreased linearly, producing a "sawtooth" shaped spectral waveform as shown below.

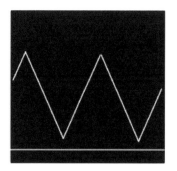 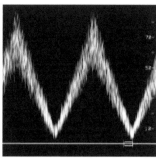

Figure 8.10 (b) (Left) Since this is an artificial target having just a single velocity, we would expect to see a single Doppler shift frequency at each instant in the spectral display. (Right) Instead we see a considerable range of frequencies caused by intrinsic spectral broadening.

Given the ideal nature of the moving object in Figure 8.10 it is clear that it must be the measurement process itself that is causing the spectral broadening seen in the display, hence the use of the term "intrinsic".

What is the cause? As with most artifacts, the cause lies in an idealisation in how we (and the machine) think about the Doppler examination. Specifically, we think of the ultrasound beam that is used to acquire the Doppler signal as a single line of sight with a single point of origin on the face of the transducer and a single Doppler angle. (Indeed this is exactly what is displayed on the screen.)

In reality we know that a significant area on the face of the transducer (the "aperture") is used to create the beam. Transmitted ultrasound travels from all of the transducer elements in the aperture to the blood vessel and echoes return to all of these elements.

Thus the Doppler signal is acquired by ultrasound travelling along a multiplicity of paths, as shown in Figure 8.11. For each of these paths the Doppler angle is different and so there will be a different Doppler shift. The overall Doppler signal will contain a mix of all these Doppler shifts.

What factors will affect the amount of spectral broadening?

- The larger the transducer aperture the worse the broadening will be. This is unfortunate, since a large aperture is needed to produce a highly focussed beam. Most ultrasound machines therefore compromise and use a smaller aperture to produce the Doppler beam than they use for grey scale imaging. This reduces intrinsic spectral broadening, but at the cost of a larger beamwidth and hence poorer spatial resolution; this is considered a reasonable price to pay for reducing the spectral broadening.

- The depth of the sample volume. The spectral broadening will be worst for superficial vessels, such as are encountered in peripheral and carotid studies.

- The Doppler angle. As we saw earlier in this chapter, variations in the angle have a more pronounced effect for large angles and a minimal effect when the angle is close to zero. Thus it should be no surprise that intrinsic spectral broadening is minimal when the Doppler angle is 0° and becomes worse as the angle increases.

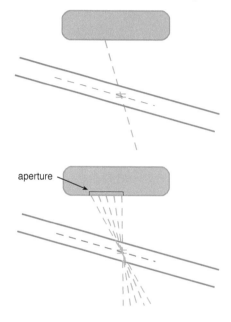

Figure 8.11 (Top) Generally we think of the Doppler beam as a single line of sight as shown here, in which case it has a single point of origin on the transducer face and a single well-defined Doppler angle. (Bottom) The reality is more complex, with multiple pathways for the ultrasound travelling to and from the transducer.

Why does this artifact matter? There are two problems that occur as a result of intrinsic spectral broadening. First, intrinsic spectral broadening causes a systematic error in every measurement of blood velocity, as shown in Figure 8.12. The more pronounced the spectral broadening is, the more the blood velocity will be overestimated.

While it may be tempting to think that the user could guess how much broadening there is and make an allowance for it when placing the measurement cursor, this is not realistic with real blood flow signals.

Secondly, spectral broadening is an important diagnostic sign. As discussed above, the Doppler signal from a blood vessel has a range of frequencies due to the fact that the sample volume contains a range of blood velocities.

In the presence of disease the range of blood velocities can increase (particularly when the blood flow becomes turbulent) and the spectrum will then have a wider range of Doppler shifts than would be found in a normal vessel. Intrinsic spectral broadening may mask or mimic the spectral broadening due to disease.

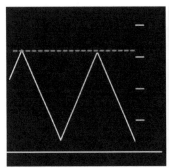 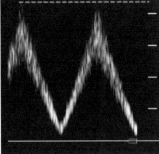

Figure 8.12 Measurements made from the spectral display will systematically overestimate the blood velocity or Doppler shift. In this example the peak velocity is overestimated by 37%.

Spectral mirror artifact

This term describes a symmetrical spectral Doppler display, as shown in Figure 8.13, with equal displacements above and below the baseline.

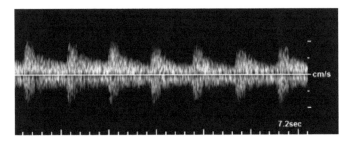

Figure 8.13 A typical example of the spectral mirror artifact.

The artifact normally occurs when the Doppler angle is 90° (see Figure 8.14). The Doppler equation predicts that there should be no Doppler signal at all in this situation, since cos 90° = 0.

What causes these artifactual signals? The answer has two parts. First, it is indeed true that there is no *real* Doppler shift. Secondly, even though there is no real Doppler shift, *intrinsic spectral broadening* still occurs, causing symmetrical spreading of the Doppler signal above and below the baseline. Figure 8.14 shows the geometry for this situation.

Thus, the signal displayed in the spectral mirror artifact is entirely artifactual; it is in fact a special case of intrinsic spectral broadening.

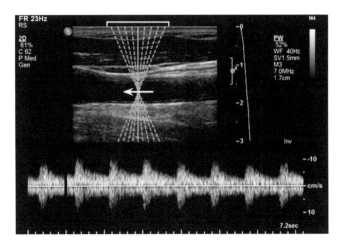

Figure 8.14 The various paths followed by the ultrasound as it travels from the probe to the sample volume and back to the probe are symmetrically placed either side of a line perpendicular to the vessel. The machine therefore "sees" identical flow towards and away from the probe.

Mirror image artifact

This artifact was described earlier in chapter 6. If a blood vessel happens to lie in tissues that are mirror-imaged, the vessel will also be duplicated and so it will appear in the mirror image.

What about blood within the vessel? Not surprisingly, the echoes from blood will also be mirror-imaged. Thus mirror-imaged vessels can be interrogated with Doppler and they will yield Doppler signals, just as they would normally. Figure 8.15 demonstrates this.

Other spectral Doppler artifacts

As with grey scale imaging, incorrect setting of the machine's controls can cause Doppler information to be lost and/or misleading appearances to be produced.

For example, if the cutoff frequency of the wall filter is set too low, Doppler shifted signals caused by wall movement will be displayed, as shown in Figure 8.16. This artifact is called "wall thump".

It is important to realise that the solution to this problem is *not* to set the wall filter cutoff very high. This would cause unnecessary loss of low velocity information from the spectral waveform as shown in Figure 8.17.

In some clinical situations the end-diastolic velocity in an artery is low or even zero, and it can be very important to determine just what its value is. Thus it is important to retain as much low velocity information as possible without introducing unacceptable wall-thump artifact.

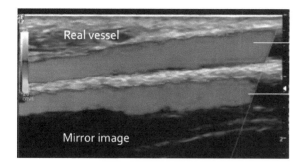

Figure 8.15 (a) This blood vessel has been mirror-imaged due to its highly reflective rear wall. The presence of flow signals in both the real vessel and the mirror image is confirmed by the colour Doppler display.

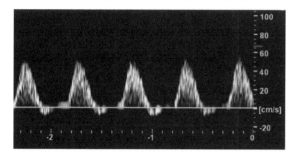

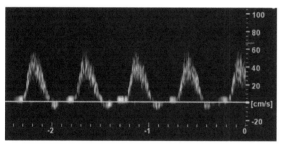

Figure 8.15 (b) Virtually identical waveforms have been acquired from the real vessel (top) and the mirror image of the vessel (bottom).

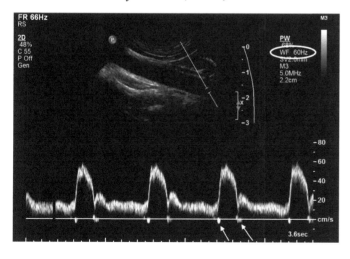

Figure 8.16 Wall thump caused by an inappropriately low setting (60 Hz) of the wall filter. The wall thump (arrows) coincides with the start and end of systole, the times when the vessel walls are moving most rapidly.

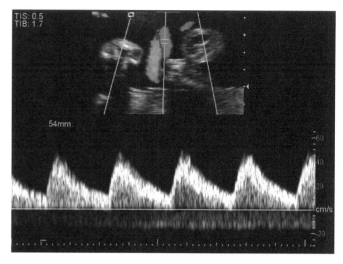

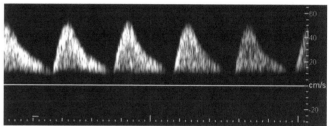

Figure 8.17 (Top) When the Doppler shift falls close to zero in diastole, as it does in this umbilical artery waveform, the wall filter cutoff must be kept low to avoid losing information. (Bottom) If the cutoff is too high it is impossible to determine the value of the end diastolic velocity.

Improper placement of the sample volume (e.g. adjacent to a vessel wall rather than in the centre of the vessel) can alter the Doppler waveform significantly, as shown in Figure 8.18.

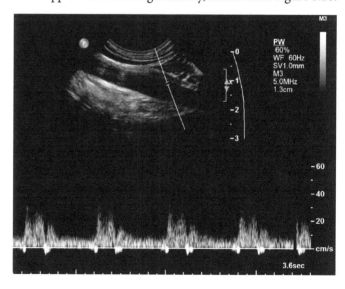

Figure 8.18 Positioning the sample volume adjacent to one wall of the vessel produces a very different Doppler waveform to that which would have been acquired from the centre of the vessel.

Similarly, using a larger than usual sample volume can produce misleading appearances as shown in Figure 8.19, since a wider range of blood velocities will contribute to the signal than when a small sample volume is used.

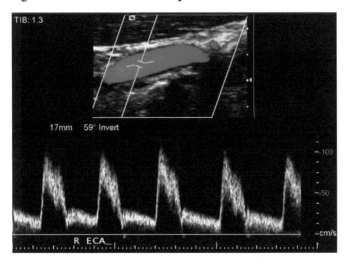

Figure 8.19 (a) When the sample volume is small relative to the vessel diameter the spectrum features a clear black "window", particularly during systole.

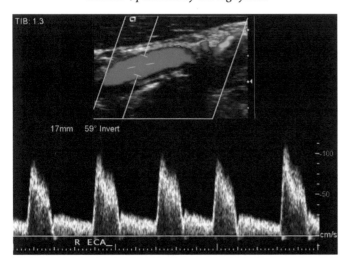

Figure 8.19 (b) If the sample volume length is made larger (in this example it spans the full width of the vessel) the spectrum is far more "filled in" than in Figure 8.19 (a).

Inappropriate settings of the Doppler gain will also cause problems as shown in Figure 8.20.

Two other important controls are the velocity scale and baseline shifting.

Both must be appropriately set to acquire useful Doppler waveforms, as shown in Figure 8.21. Thus all of these controls – Doppler gain, wall filter cutoff, sample volume size and location, velocity scale and baseline position – must be properly set for valid and useful Doppler waveforms to be acquired.

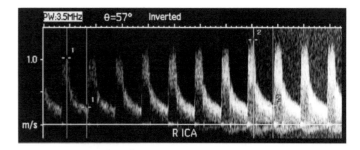

Figure 8.20 In this acquisition, the Doppler gain was increased as the display swept across the screen. On the left the gain is too low, and the peak velocity will be underestimated. On the right the gain is too high, causing overestimation of the velocity and a "snowstorm" effect due to electronic noise.

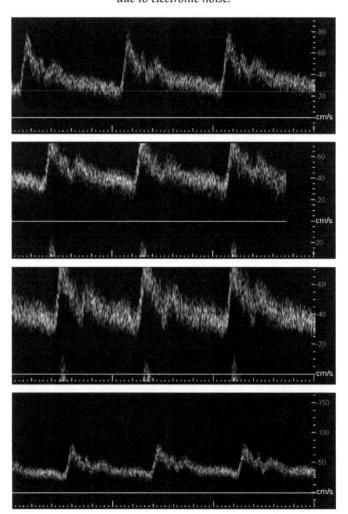

Figure 8.21 Internal carotid artery waveforms showing: (a) appropriate settings of the velocity scale and baseline, with the waveform filling most of the available display range; (b) the baseline is too high, causing aliasing to become visible; (c) the velocity scale is too low causing aliasing; (d) the velocity scale is too high so the waveform is small and cannot be seen well or measured accurately.

Lastly, what about electrical interference?

Since Doppler systems are very sensitive (due to the low level of the echoes from blood), they are particularly susceptible to electrical interference.

Typically this will produce "snowstorm" or "cobweb" or other appearances in the spectral display which can be readily distinguished from real Doppler information.

Suggested activities

1. Set the spectral baseline in the centre (i.e. with equal display range above and below the line). Acquire an arterial Doppler waveform, then decrease the velocity scale until aliasing occurs. Move the baseline to remove the effect of the aliasing.

2. Try to produce a spectral mirror artifact (as shown in Figure 8.14) by arranging for the Doppler beam to be at 90° to a vessel.

3. Experiment with the size and positioning of the sample volume while acquiring Doppler signals from an artery. Observe the effect on the Doppler spectral display.

4. Vary the Doppler gain and wall filter settings. Again, observe the effect on the spectrum as you alter these controls.

Colour Doppler artifacts

Most colour Doppler artifacts are unique, though some are related to artifacts we have already seen with grey scale imaging and/or pulsed Doppler.

Colour aliasing

Aliasing is one of the most important artifacts in colour Doppler. It causes an abrupt reversal in colour suggesting incorrectly that the direction of flow has changed (see Figure 8.22).

How can we determine that this appearance is due to aliasing and that it is not a genuine difference in flow direction?

Two tests can be applied. The first requires the user to carefully examine the region in the vessel where the colour changes abruptly (circled). If the colours in adjacent pixels change from orange to blue-green (colours representing the maximum detectable Doppler shifts in each direction) then it must be aliasing. If there was a genuine change in flow direction the adjacent red and blue areas would be dark red and dark blue, representing low Doppler shifts close to the baseline.

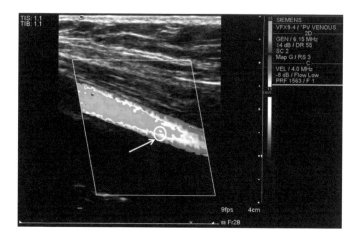

Figure 8.22 (a) In the central part of this artery there is a blue-green "island" surrounded by red and orange. While this suggests that the flow is reversed in the centre of the vessel, in fact it is caused by aliasing.

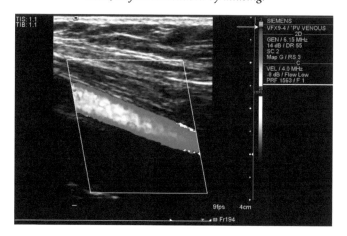

Figure 8.22 (b) The colour baseline has been shifted (arrow) so that almost all the display range is in the red direction. The aliasing has been eliminated.

The second test will be familiar from spectral Doppler. The colour baseline can be moved. If, as the baseline shifts the blue-green colour is steadily reduced (and perhaps eliminated) then it was aliasing.

Figure 8.22 shows the use of baseline shifting to eliminate aliasing.

Note that in some situations colour aliasing is seen as a useful artifact since it highlights areas with high Doppler shift.

Colour dropout

Sometimes colour is not displayed when it should be.

There are a number of possible causes for this. The Doppler signal may be too weak to detect because the vessel is small and/or because it is deep in the body. Alternatively, the colour Doppler settings may not have been optimised.

Figure 8.23 (a) shows an example of dropout caused by inappropriate instrument settings.

When the colour gain is increased as shown in Figure 8.23 (b), the vessel is completely filled with colour as would be expected.

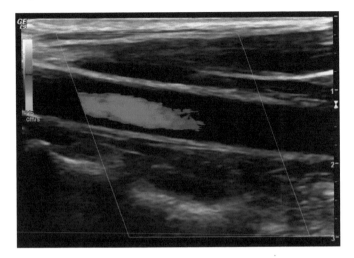

Figure 8.23 (a) The colour Doppler in this common carotid artery only partially fills the vessel due to inadequate colour Doppler gain. In particular, the slower moving blood near the vessel walls has not been detected.

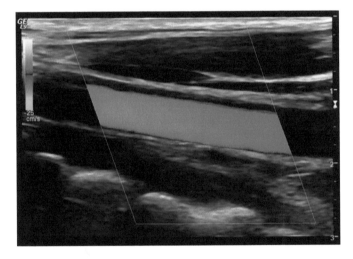

Figure 8.23 (b) Increasing the colour Doppler gain has eliminated the problem and the vessel is filled with colour.

What can be done to improve the detection of flow? Clearly the user should make sure that the machine has been optimised for the specific vessel(s) that they are trying to visualise.

Actions that should be taken include:

- Check that an appropriate preset has been used (e.g. that you have not chosen an arterial preset when you are trying to image veins).
- Try increasing the colour gain.

- Reduce the probe frequency, since this will reduce tissue attenuation.
- Try reducing the cutoff frequency of the wall filter, since it may be suppressing low Doppler-shift signals from slow-moving blood.
- Try increasing the grey-scale priority, since the tissue/blood discrimination function may be suppressing colour in areas where there are low-level grey scale artifacts.
- Try reducing the colour velocity scale. If the velocity scale is too high then signals from slow-moving blood will not be detected.
- Check that the Doppler angle is not close to 90°, since this will make the Doppler shift too low to detect. If the angle is too large, reduce it by steering the colour box or by moving the probe.
- Try using power mode colour Doppler, since it is significantly more sensitive that standard colour Doppler, as explained in chapter 7.
- Consider increasing the transmit power if it is possible to do so safely.

Colour bleed

Sometimes the opposite to dropout occurs – colour information is displayed where it should not be (see Figure 8.24).

To eliminate colour bleeding:

- Check that an appropriate preset has been selected for the examination.
- Reduce the grey-sale priority setting; if it is too high then tissue echoes will not suppress the colour information when they should.
- Increase the wall-filter cutoff frequency.
- Try reducing the colour gain.
- Check that the colour velocity scale is set appropriately.

Angle effects

The Doppler shift detected, and therefore the colour displayed, at each point in a colour Doppler image is determined by both the blood velocity and the Doppler angle at that point.

In this way colour Doppler is no different to pulsed and CW Doppler. What is different about colour is that it is not generally feasible to apply angle correction to the image. With both curved and phased array probes the method used to scan the beam means that *every beam has a different direction and therefore a different Doppler angle.*

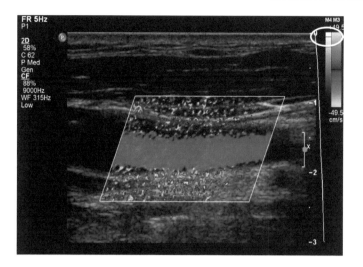

Figure 8.24 (a) An example of colour "bleeding", where colour is wrongly displayed outside the blood vessel. In this case it has occurred because the grey scale priority has been set much higher than normal (as shown by the horizontal line on the grey scale bar to the left of the colour bar, circled).

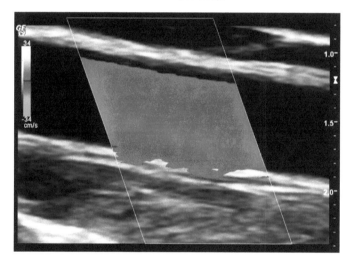

Figure 8.24 (b) A second example of colour bleeding, in this case due to excessively high colour gain. Once again, this is likely to indicate that the colour Doppler settings have not been optimised for the vessel(s) under study.

Thus, even when the vessel(s) under study are straight, the Doppler angle will vary across the image, as shown in Figures 8.25 and 8.26 (a). In addition, it is not uncommon for vessels to curve, as shown in Figure 8.26 (b), further complicating the issue.

These examples show situations where the angle effect is quite obvious.

Often, however, the effect is more subtle, and it is not uncommon for users to mistakenly interpret changes in colour caused by changes in angle as being due to changes in velocity.

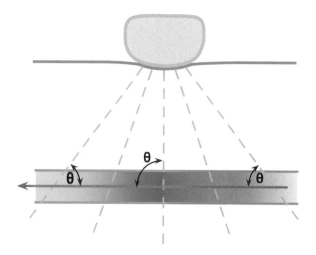

Figure 8.25 With curved and phased arrays every beam is directed at a different angle relative to the probe. A range of colours will therefore be seen even in the simplest case of a straight vessel with uniform flow velocity.

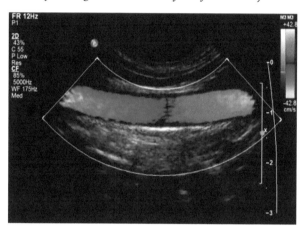

Figure 8.26 (a) A clinical example of a straight vessel imaged using a curved array probe. The variation in colour is entirely due to the change in Doppler angle as the beam sweeps through the field of view (see Figure 8.25).

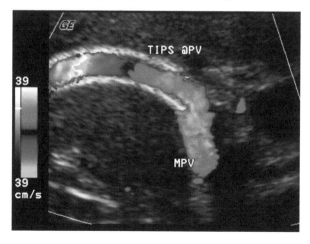

Figure 8.26 (b) In a curved vessel the Doppler angle will vary along the length of the vessel, no matter what type of probe is used, and so the colours will vary continually.

This important point is worth repeating. Colour Doppler should be viewed as being a qualitative modality, complementary to pulsed and CW Doppler. The latter are capable of providing objective quantitative information.

Mirror image

As we have seen, this is a common artifact in ultrasound imaging. A strongly reflective interface acts like a mirror, causing superficial tissues to be replicated as a mirror image deep to the interface. If the region that is being mirror-imaged contains blood vessels, they will be displayed in the mirror image too. The echoes from the blood are mirror-imaged in the same way as the tissue echoes and so Doppler signals can be obtained from the mirror images of the vessels, as shown in Figure 8.15.

Depending on the orientation of the reflective interface producing the mirror image, the flow in the mirror image may be in the same direction as in the true image of the vessel or it may be in the opposite direction.

Twinkle artifact

Small calcified and crystalline structures can produce echoes which mimic movement, producing a characteristic appearance in the colour Doppler display (see Figure 8.27). A mixture of red and blue colours is typically seen, fluctuating in time. The artifact is therefore termed the "twinkle artifact". Like shadowing and enhancement in grey scale images, this appearance can be a useful sign of the presence of small calcifications and similar materials.

Suggested activities

1. Acquire a colour Doppler image from an artery. Make sure the colour baseline is in the centre of the colour bar. Reduce the colour velocity scale until the image shows aliasing. Shift the baseline to eliminate the aliasing again.

2. Again acquire a colour Doppler image in an artery. Increase the colour velocity scale and watch for any colour dropout. Note particularly whether the dropout occurs at the edges of the vessel and in the diastolic phase of the heart cycle.

3. Obtain a colour Doppler image in an artery such as the common carotid or the femoral artery. Without altering the controls, move the transducer to image an adjacent vein. Adjust the steering if necessary to ensure the angle is similar. Note whether the colour is well displayed in the vein, or whether you need to readjust the velocity scale to optimise the image.

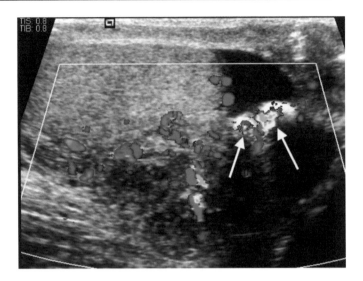

Figure 8.27 (a) An example of twinkle artifact caused by scrotoliths (free floating calcific entities often found in the scrotum). In real time the artifact "twinkles" red and blue which differentiates it from the colour in blood vessels.

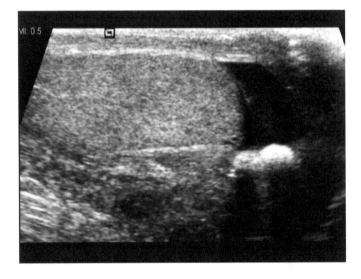

Figure 8.27 (b) In this image the scrotoliths are clearly visible as echogenic foci.

Chapter 9
Haemodynamic concepts

Cardiovascular system

The cardiovascular system is very simple if we look at the big picture. The heart is simply a pump which has the job of circulating blood around a closed loop of blood vessels.

Looking in more detail (see Figure 9.1), we can see that blood travels from the heart through arteries which branch to form smaller arteries, then to arterioles (very small arteries). From here the blood goes to the capillaries where it delivers oxygen and nutrients to the tissues and transfers waste products. It then travels through venules (very small veins) which combine to form larger veins, then back to the heart.

Doppler ultrasound is a very valuable diagnostic technique for detecting and quantifying disease of most of the elements of this system – the heart, arteries and veins. Doppler can also be used to detect abnormalities in organ function if they affect blood flow patterns. It can also be used to assess the perfusion of a region, whether it be the normal circulation within an organ or abnormal circulation associated with a lesion.

To understand how Doppler is used to make these diagnoses, it is necessary to understand some basic principles of blood flow dynamics.

Blood flow and blood pressure

The heart creates relatively high blood pressure in the major arteries, while the pressure in the veins is far lower. It is this pressure difference between the arteries and veins that causes blood to circulate throughout the body. In this section we will look at the relationship between blood flow (the volume of blood that travels through a given part of the circulation) and the arterial-venous pressure difference.

An important observation is that different regions (e.g. the brain and the arms) may see exactly the same arterial-venous pressure difference but the volume of blood flow through them may be very different (see Figure 9.2).

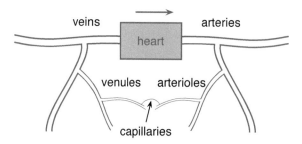

Figure 9.1 The basic elements of the cardiovascular system.

The brain demands a high blood flow at all times, whereas the arms require relatively little flow, especially when not exercising. How can this happen?

The answer lies in what is termed the "flow resistance" of each of these circulations.

A high resistance circulation like the arms at rest requires relatively little blood whereas a low resistance circulation like the brain demands a high flow rate.

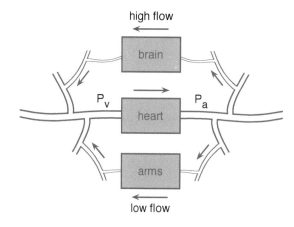

Figure 9.2 The blood supply for both the brain and the arms originates close to the heart, so the arterio-venous pressure difference applied to them (P_a - P_v) is essentially the same, yet the amount of blood flow through them is very different.

Mathematically the relationship between flow, pressure and resistance is expressed as follows:

$$Q = \frac{P_a - P_v}{R}$$

where Q is the mean or average flow rate (expressed in ml/min or l/min), P_a and P_v are the mean arterial and venous pressures respectively and R is the flow resistance of the circulation.

What determines the resistance and why does it vary from one part of the body to another?

While all of the vessels in a given organ or body region contribute to its resistance, the dominant factor is the number and the diameter of the arterioles. These small arteries are often termed "resistance vessels" for this reason. The larger they are and the more of them there are, the lower the resistance will be. The other important variable is whether vessels are "in parallel" or "in series" (see Figure 9.3).

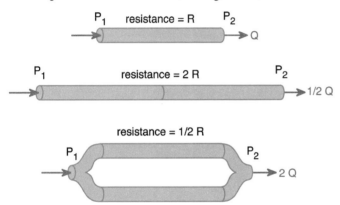

Figure 9.3 (Top) A single blood vessel carries a flow Q and has a flow resistance of R. (Centre) Placing two of these vessels "in series" doubles the resistance and therefore halves the flow. (Bottom) If instead two vessels are placed "in parallel" then they carry twice as much flow as the single vessel and so the resistance has been halved. (Note the pressures are the same in each case.) A low resistance circulation will have a large number of vessels in parallel.

A second important observation is that the blood flow to many organs and body regions changes depending on need. Blood flow to the limbs (and other muscles) increases with exercise. Similarly blood flow to the gastrointestinal tract increases substantially after a meal, and flow to the uterus increases dramatically in pregnancy.

How can the body alter the resistance of the circulation in a given region? The answer is that the arterioles are capable of opening and closing. When more flow is needed, many more arterioles are opened up and flow increases. (Think of the way your face gets flushed when you are hot. This is caused by the opening up of additional vessels in the superficial tissues to help the body get rid of the excess heat.)

In some situations new blood vessels are formed. This is termed "neovascularisation" and it is characteristic of malignancies, where the new blood vessels support the rapid growth that is typical of malignant tissue.

In this section we have been looking at *blood flow* and *blood pressure*. However, remember that Doppler ultrasound gives us information about *blood velocity*, that is the speed at which the blood is flowing, not the rate of flow. We will therefore need to examine how disease affects blood velocity.

Stenotic disease

A major type of vascular disease is stenosis, that is an abnormal narrowing of a vessel. (Heart valves can also become stenosed.) A common cause of vascular stenosis is atherosclerosis which typically causes a localised narrowing of the affected vessel. In time the narrowing grows more severe and it can eventually lead to complete occlusion, that is blocking of the vessel.

Often stenosis affects the larger arteries supplying blood to a given region. Typical sites include the carotid artery (supplying blood to the brain), brachial arteries (supplying blood to the arms), iliac and femoral arteries (supplying blood to the legs) and renal arteries (supplying blood to the kidneys).

In the earlier stages of the disease the effect of a stenosis on blood flow will be negligible and it may be quite asymptomatic and therefore go undetected. As it becomes more severe it will reach the point where it becomes a "critical" or "haemodynamically significant" stenosis. At this stage blood flow to the organ or region is reduced. As the narrowing becomes more severe flow is reduced further, eventually stopping when the vessel is totally occluded. Clearly haemodynamically significant disease is likely to cause symptoms (e.g. leg pain with exercise).

Even though minor to moderate stenosis will have little effect on blood flow, it can subject the patient to the risk of an embolus – a small piece of tissue, blood clot or other material which breaks away from the stenosis and travels along the artery until it becomes wedged in a small vessel. Carotid artery stenosis, for example, is associated with an increased likelihood of stroke.

It is therefore clear that we want to detect stenotic disease as early as possible and to estimate its severity, usually expressed as the percentage reduction in the cross-sectional area (or diameter) of the artery. In some patients we may also want to track the disease over time to follow its progression.

How can we do this if mild to moderate stenosis generally has little or no effect on the rate of flow in the artery? The answer lies in *localised* changes to the blood velocity caused by the stenosis. Thus an examination aimed at determining if a patient has renal artery stenosis will involve scanning the *entire length* of both the main renal arteries using Doppler to search for localised changes to the blood velocity.

What are these changes to the blood velocity? Figure 9.4 (a) shows the main effect of stenosis. The blood velocity must increase to compensate for the narrowing of the vessel.

Clearly this is ideally suited to detection by Doppler, since it will lead to increased Doppler shifts from within the narrowed area of the vessel and immediately beyond it.

Figure 9.4 (b) shows a second effect. Immediately downstream from the stenosis the blood must slow down again since the vessel has returned to its normal diameter.

This creates vortices (resembling small whirlpools in the blood) and, if the stenosis is severe, chaotic flow (referred to as turbulence). In either case the result is a wider range of Doppler shifts than would normally be detected. This is termed spectral broadening (see Figure 9.5).

Thus the typical Doppler signs of stenotic disease are:

- increased blood velocity within and immediately downstream from the affected area, and
- spectral broadening in the immediate post-stenotic portion of the vessel.

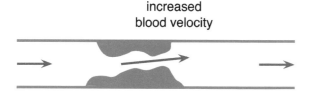

Figure 9.4 (a) As the blood enters the stenotic (narrowed) section of the vessel it accelerates. The increase in the blood velocity can be readily detected by Doppler within and immediately beyond the stenosis.

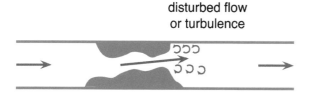

Figure 9.4 (b) The jet of fast-moving blood must slow down as it emerges from the stenosis. This leads to the formation of eddies (small whirlpools) or even chaotic turbulence. The result is an increase in the range of Doppler shifts from the region, i.e. spectral broadening.

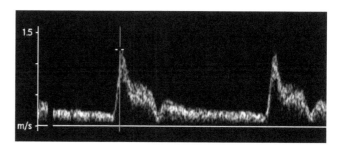

Figure 9.5 (a) The waveform from a healthy vessel shows a relatively narrow spectrum.

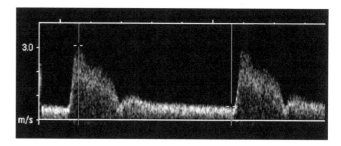

Figure 9.5 (b) The waveform immediately distal to a stenosis shows increased velocities and obvious spectral broadening, with the Doppler signal "filled in" all the way to the baseline and even extending below the baseline.

Note that the fast-moving jet of blood passing through the narrowed area may be directed at an angle (as shown in Figure 9.4), not parallel to the vessel walls. In this case colour Doppler can be useful to determine the direction of flow to allow more accurate angle correction and therefore more accurate measurement of the blood velocity.

As the disease becomes more severe these changes become more pronounced. This means we can estimate the percentage stenosis from measurements of the increased velocity and spectral broadening. Specific diagnostic criteria have been developed for each of the arteries commonly affected by stenotic disease. These criteria are generally based on the increased blood velocity values (usually peak systolic and minimum or end diastolic velocities) and the degree of spectral broadening.

Velocity waveform

So far we have discussed the measurement of specific velocity values from the Doppler spectral display (e.g. peak systolic and minimum or end diastolic velocities) and their use in the diagnosis of stenosis.

Now we will consider another major feature of the Doppler spectrum, the velocity waveform. This refers to the shape traced out over time by the Doppler signal.

Earlier in this chapter we considered two different circulations – the brain and the arms – which derive their blood flow from approximately the same point in the cardiovascular system. We saw that the rates of flow through them are very different, even though the driving force applied to them (the arterial-venous pressure difference) is essentially the same. We noted that this is due to the difference in the resistance of the two circulations, and that this reflects differences in the amount of flow required by each region.

When arterial waveforms from these two circulations are compared it is clear that they too are very different. Indeed, each major artery tends to have its own distinctive waveform "signature". Importantly, the shape of the waveform in each artery is determined largely by the resistance of the region to which it is supplying blood (see Figures 9.6 and 9.7).

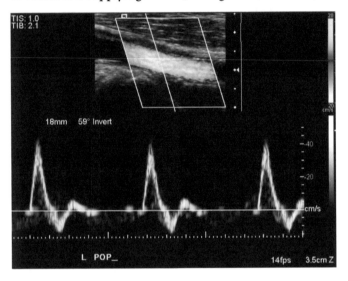

Figure 9.6 (a) A typical high resistance arterial waveform, in this case from the popliteal artery in a subject who is resting.

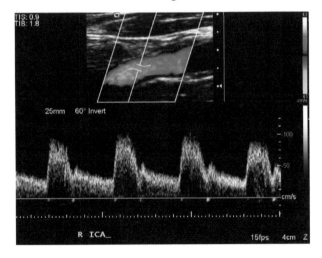

Figure 9.6 (b) A typical low resistance arterial waveform from the internal carotid artery.

High resistance circulations (like the limbs at rest) display highly pulsatile waveforms, as shown in Figure 9.6 (a). The main features are rapid acceleration and deceleration at the start and end of systole, a brief reversal of the direction of flow at the start of diastole and then little or no flow for the rest of the diastolic phase.

Low resistance circulations (like the brain) display less pulsatile waveforms as shown in Figure 9.6 (b). The main features are the absence of any flow reversal and sustained flow throughout the diastolic period. (Note that when the word "pulsatile" is used to describe waveforms it refers to the amount of variation of the velocity in each heart cycle.)

This relationship between the arterial waveform and the resistance of the circulation that the artery is supplying with blood suggests that there must be a "normal" waveform for each artery. Further, it suggests that when the waveform in a given artery is markedly different to what is expected it must mean there is an abnormality or a change in functional status.

As an example, Doppler signals can be readily acquired from the fetus during pregnancy, and in many centres Doppler has become a routine part of obstetric examinations. Doppler signals can be obtained from vessels such as the umbilical artery and the fetal renal and cerebral arteries. Deviations from normal waveforms are indicative of problems such as intrauterine growth restriction.

A second example is when Doppler is used to examine a transplant kidney to determine whether it is being adequately perfused with blood.

Waveforms acquired from arteries throughout the renal tissues are compared with the expected waveform shape. Abnormal waveforms are suggestive of vascular problems and/or transplant rejection.

How are arterial waveforms assessed? It is possible to simply describe their main features – the speed of acceleration and deceleration, whether or not there is flow reversal in diastole, the amount of diastolic flow etc. However, it is clearly desirable to have one or more numerical measures that allow waveforms to be characterised and compared more objectively with normal waveforms.

A number of indices based on measurements of Doppler shift (or velocity) are used for this purpose. Figure 9.7 shows waveforms derived by tracing the outlines of the spectral tracings in Figure 9.6. The definitions of the specific Doppler values used to calculate the most widely used indices are also shown.

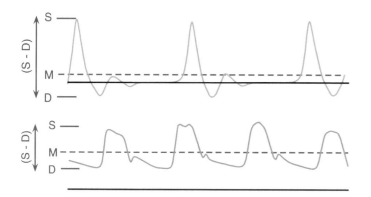

Figure 9.7 Waveforms obtained by tracing the envelope (i.e. the upper edge) of the Doppler spectral tracings shown in Figure 9.6. S is the peak systolic velocity, D is the minimum diastolic velocity and M is the mean (i.e. the average) velocity over a heart cycle.

The most commonly used indices are the Resistance Index (RI), the Pulsatility Index (PI) and the Systolic/Diastolic Ratio (S/D), defined as follows:

$$RI = \frac{(S-D)}{S}$$

$$PI = \frac{(S-D)}{M}$$

$$S/D = \frac{S}{D}$$

S is the peak systolic velocity, D is the lowest diastolic velocity and M is the mean velocity over an entire cardiac cycle.

The quantity (S - D) is simply the overall range of values from maximum to minimum (see Figure 9.7). Note that (S - D) is larger for the high resistance waveform (upper trace) than for the low resistance waveform (lower trace). The numerical values of the indices calculated from these two waveforms are as follows.

Upper waveform (popliteal artery):

RI = 1.2

PI = 9.6

S/D = -4.4

Lower waveform (internal carotid artery):

RI = 0.67

PI = 1.1

S/D = 3.0

Note that both the Resistance and Pulsatility indices are substantially higher for the high resistance popliteal artery waveform, as we would expect.

Note also that the S/D ratio for the popliteal artery has changed sign (i.e. it is negative) due to the fact that the minimum diastolic velocity is in the opposite direction to the systolic velocity.

What would happen if the minimum diastolic velocity was zero? The S/D ratio would then become infinite, highlighting the fact that it is not a good choice of index for most purposes. In contrast, both the RI and PI are useful regardless of whether the minimum diastolic velocity is forward, reversed or zero.

How does the Doppler angle affect these waveform indices? If we consider the Doppler measurements shown in Figure 9.7 (S, D and M) we recognise that all of them are proportional to $\cos \theta$ where θ is the Doppler angle. Since all of the indices are calculated as ratios of Doppler shifts, the $\cos \theta$ factor cancels out, making the indices *independent of the Doppler angle*.

Thus we should expect to get the same value for these indices regardless of the Doppler angle used (as long as it is not close to 90°) and regardless of whether we have angle corrected or not. We would even expect to get the same values for the indices if we were to use CW Doppler to acquire the signals.

Velocity profile

In order to better understand what Doppler signals can tell us about the circulation, we have looked at the localised effects of stenosis on blood velocity. We have also looked at the concept of flow resistance and how resistance affects arterial waveforms.

In this section we will look at another detail of blood flow – the way the blood velocity varies across a vessel's diameter. This is called the velocity profile.

The term "laminar flow" is used to describe smooth stable flow. Figure 9.8 shows the parabolic velocity profile found in laminar flow. This name comes from the fact that the profile can be described mathematically as a parabola.

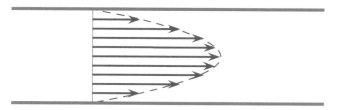

Figure 9.8 For laminar flow in a straight vessel the velocity profile is parabolic.

The major features of this profile are that the velocity is fastest in the centre of the vessel and decreases steadily as we move away from the centre towards the edges of the vessel.

Adjacent to the vessel walls the blood is moving very slowly. Also notice that flow is directly along the vessel, parallel to the vessel walls.

Why does this velocity profile occur? The answer is that it is due to friction. As blood moves along the vessel there is friction between it and the vessel walls. This tends to slow down the "boundary layer", i.e. the blood immediately adjacent to the walls. The boundary layer therefore moves much more slowly than the blood in the centre of the vessel.

There are also friction forces within fluids. Thus the slow-moving boundary layer tends to slow down the blood adjacent to it. That blood in turn slows the layer of blood adjacent to it, and so on.

As we move from the walls towards the centre of the vessel we therefore find that the blood velocity progressively increases until we reach the centre of the vessel where it is at a maximum (see Figure 9.9).

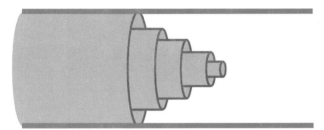

Figure 9.9 It can be useful to think of flowing blood as a series of layers (laminae), each moving at a different speed. Friction forces mean that slower moving blood tends to slow down the faster moving blood adjacent to it. The overall result is the parabolic profile.

What are the implications of the parabolic velocity profile for Doppler measurements? Figure 9.10 shows two possible situations, depending on the size of the sample volume relative to the vessel. A given clinical situation may resemble one or other of these situations, or it may fall somewhere in between, as shown in Figures 9.11 and 9.12.

Is the profile always parabolic? No, whenever the flow in a vessel is disturbed the velocity profile changes. There are many situations where this can happen, for example:

- when the vessel is curved;
- when the vessel branches;
- when the vessel is significantly stenotic;
- when the blood is strongly accelerated or decelerated.

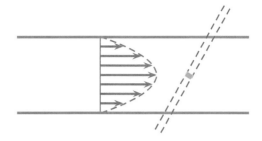

Figure 9.10 (a) When the sample volume is small compared with the vessel and it is positioned in the centre of the vessel, a limited range of velocities will be "seen" and so the Doppler spectrum will be relatively narrow.

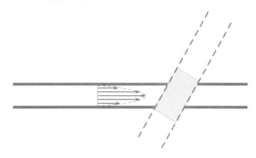

Figure 9.10 (b) Conversely, if the vessel is so small that it lies completely within the sample volume, the full range of velocities from zero to maximum will be seen and the Doppler signal will be uniformly filled in to the baseline.

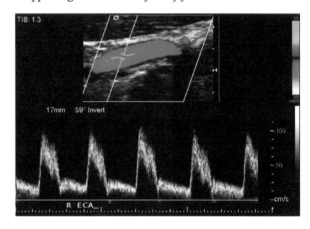

Figure 9.11 (a) Normal spectral waveform showing a relatively narrow spectrum with a clear "window" under the spectrum.

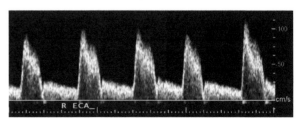

Figure 9.11 (b) The sample volume has been increased in size so that it spans the entire width of the vessel. This has caused the spectrum to fill in, mimicking the effects of spectral broadening.

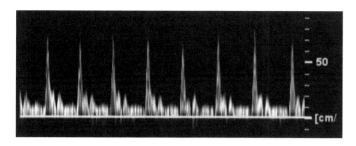

Figure 9.12. This radial artery waveform is relatively broad (i.e. filled in) due to the small size of the vessel relative to the beam and sample volume.

A dramatic example of flow that is not parallel to the vessel walls is shown in Figure 9.13. When blood travels around a curved section of vessel it follows a helical path, corkscrewing as it travels around the curve.

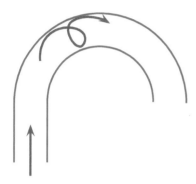

Figure 9.13 When the blood is forced around a curved section of vessel like the aortic arch it follows a helical flow pattern.

Depending on the geometry of the vessel and the speed of flow, a phenomenon known as "boundary layer separation" may also occur, as shown in Figure 9.14. Here the blood adjacent to the wall (the boundary layer) has failed to negotiate a sharp bend and it has separated from the wall, causing a localised area of swirling blood to form.

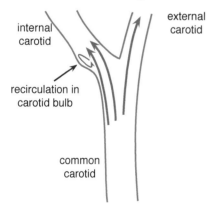

Figure 9.14 In some situations the boundary layer fails to stay in contact with the wall as the blood rounds a sharp curve such as the carotid bifurcation. Boundary layer separation then occurs, leading to an area of recirculation.

Boundary layer separation is routinely seen in the carotid bifurcation, where the common carotid artery divides into the internal and external carotid arteries, with recirculation being seen in the carotid bulb.

What happens downstream from a disturbance such as a curve, branch or diseased portion of vessel? The parabolic profile gradually reasserts itself and flow returns to the normal laminar pattern.

What happens when the blood is strongly accelerated or decelerated, e.g. at the beginning and end of systole?

A phenomenon known as "plug flow" occurs. As shown in Figure 9.15, the velocity profile is flat, i.e. the blood has the same velocity at all points across the vessel's diameter. The result will be an unusually narrow Doppler spectrum since all the blood is travelling at the same velocity. Again, this effect is short-lived and the profile quickly returns to parabolic.

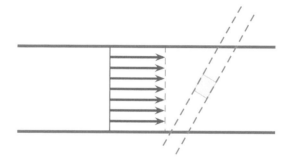

Figure 9.15 With strong acceleration (or deceleration) the profile flattens. The range of velocities seen in the Doppler sample volume is then narrower than usual.

Venous disease

As discussed earlier, the veins return blood to the heart. Blood flow in veins may be driven by pulsatile pressure from the heart (as seen in the cerebral circulation), but often other factors are important. When walking, for example, the rhythmic compression of the leg muscles drives venous blood from the legs back up to the heart. This is known as the "muscle pump". Similarly, rhythmic variation of the pressure in the chest due to breathing can drive venous flow.

These venous flow mechanisms are effective because the veins contain valves which prevent blood from flowing backwards in the veins. These valves may stop functioning properly, leading to venous "incompetence" and a variety of symptoms such as varicose veins and swelling of the legs. Spectral and colour Doppler can be used to detect the back flow through the valves.

Another important disease is venous thrombosis, where blood clots block veins and impair the circulation.

While thrombus may be visible in greyscale images it is more reliably detected using the ultrasound probe to compress the vein in question. Healthy veins will collapse under pressure from the probe while clot-filled veins will not.

As with arterial disease, this brief survey cannot do justice to the range of venous diseases and the role of ultrasound in their diagnosis.

However, a more detailed discussion is beyond the scope of this book.

Suggested activities

1. Compare arterial waveforms acquired from a range of different arteries such as the common carotid, brachial, hepatic, renal and femoral arteries. Identify which are high resistance waveforms and which are low resistance. Think about the nature of each circulation and whether you would expect it to be high or low resistance.

2. Place a small sample volume in the centre of a common carotid artery and record the Doppler spectrum. Move the sample volume to one side of the vessel and note how the spectral display changes.

3. Acquire a Doppler signal from a small artery such as the radial artery. Note whether the spectrum is more "filled in" than for a larger artery due to the fact that the sample volume is covering more of the vessel and so seeing a wider range of velocities.

Summary

In this chapter we have reviewed some of the main aspects of blood flow dynamics as they relate to Doppler diagnosis. We have seen that:

1. Arterial stenosis can be diagnosed using localised Doppler findings of increased blood velocity and spectral broadening. Measurements of these parameters allow the severity of a stenosis to be estimated.

2. Flow resistance is a useful concept relating to the amount of blood flow a given organ or body region requires.

3. The resistance of a given circulation can be inferred from the velocity waveform in the artery that supplies it with blood. Abnormalities in the waveform suggest abnormal function of the organ or body region, and can be characterised using waveform indices such as the Pulsatility Index and Resistance Index.

4. The waveform indices are independent of the Doppler angle and so they can be used even when a vessel is not visible and Doppler angle correction cannot be applied.

5. The velocity profile is parabolic in laminar flow but it changes in a number of circumstances. Since the profile affects the width of the Doppler spectrum the user must be aware of these effects.

6. Helical flow occurs in curved vessels, and boundary separation can occur in some situations. These are examples of flow conditions where the direction of flow is not parallel to the vessel walls.

7. Venous diseases such as venous incompetence and thrombosis can be diagnosed using Doppler and imaging.

Chapter 10

Equipment performance

Introductory comments

In this chapter we will review the factors that affect ultrasound image quality. We will also look at how imaging and Doppler performance can be assessed objectively.

What makes a good ultrasound image? Most experienced users of ultrasound can judge image quality, at least subjectively. However, they may not be able to explain how they make this judgement, i.e. what criteria they are using. We will look here at more objective ways of talking about image quality and what makes a good image. This will allow us to determine which equipment factors are limiting performance and what must be changed to improve the images.

Three different aspects of the image are taken into account. They are termed spatial resolution, contrast resolution and temporal resolution.

Spatial resolution

This term is used to quantify the "sharpness" of the image (i.e. its lack of blurriness).

The formal definition of spatial resolution is the minimum spacing required between two small objects (usually referred to as "point targets") so that they will be seen as separate objects in the image. If the targets are spaced more closely together than this, they will blur together and appear as a single object. We would then say that they have not been "resolved" in the image.

For ultrasound images the spatial resolution is further divided into two components – axial and lateral resolution.

Axial resolution

Axial resolution is the minimum separation in depth that is needed between two point targets lying along the same line of sight (i.e. beam direction) which allows them to be resolved in the image.

To determine the axial resolution for a given machine and probe, we need to look at the echoes received from the two point targets (see Figure 10.1). If the echoes do not overlap, the point targets will be resolved and seen as separate objects.

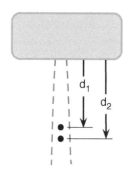

Figure 10.1 (a) Two point targets lie on the same line of sight at different depths.

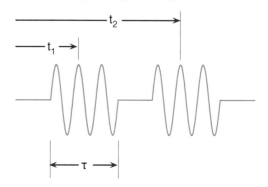

Figure 10.1 (b) The echo signal from the two point targets. As long as the echoes do not overlap the two targets will be resolved in the image.

The axial resolution is therefore the minimum separation of the point targets in depth for which the echoes do not overlap. The echoes will not overlap as long as their arrival times (t_1 and t_2) differ by at least τ, the transmit pulse duration, that is:

$$t_2 - t_1 > \tau$$

In chapter 3 we saw that there is a simple relationship between the depth of an object in the tissues (d) and the arrival time of its echo (t):

$$t = \frac{2d}{c}$$

Substituting this in the previous equation we can see that the two targets will be resolved as long as:

$$\left(\frac{2d_2}{c}\right) - \left(\frac{2d_1}{c}\right) > \tau$$

$$\frac{2(d_2 - d_1)}{c} > \tau$$

$$(d_2 - d_1) > \frac{c\tau}{2}$$

Thus we can see that the axial resolution of an ultrasound image is $(c\tau/2)$ where τ is the transmit pulse duration. The quantity $(c\tau)$ is sometimes called the "spatial pulse length", so the axial resolution is simply half the spatial pulse length.

As an example, if a machine is operating at 6 MHz and the transmit pulse contains just three cycles, the pulse duration will be 0.5 µsec and the axial resolution will be 0.39 mm.

We can therefore see that the shorter the transmit pulse duration is the better the axial resolution will be. In chapters 3 and 4 we saw that this is most readily achieved by making the ultrasound frequency as high as possible (consistent with achieving adequate depth of penetration) and by using broadband transducers.

Note that the axial resolution is independent of depth and is the same throughout the image, since the transmit pulse duration is constant. This is not true for lateral resolution.

Lateral resolution

In chapter 4 we saw that the image of an object is smeared out laterally by an amount equal to the beamwidth.

Referring to Figure 10.2, it can be readily seen that two objects at the same depth must therefore be separated by at least the beamwidth in order to be resolved. Thus the lateral resolution is simply equal to the beamwidth.

As an example, a machine operating at 6 MHz with an aperture of 2.5 cm focussed at a depth of 4 cm will have a beamwidth at focus of 1.0 mm.

How can the beamwidth (and therefore the lateral resolution) be minimised?

We saw earlier that the beamwidth is minimised by using as high a frequency as possible and as large a transducer aperture as possible.

Practical considerations such as the size of the acoustic window limit the aperture. We can therefore see that both axial and lateral resolution will be best when the highest frequency is used consistent with the required depth of penetration.

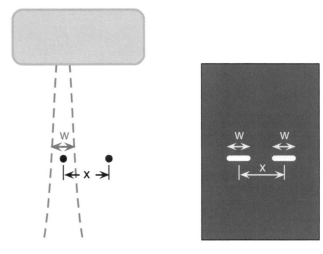

Figure 10.2 The finite width of the ultrasound beam causes a point target to be smeared out laterally in the image by an amount equal to the beamwidth (w). The separation (x) must therefore be larger than the beamwidth for the echoes to remain separate in the image.

Note that the lateral resolution will vary with depth, being best at the focal depth and worse at other depths. A practical implication of this is that *the depth of focus should be carefully adjusted so that it is placed in the region of interest.*

Note in Figure 10.3 that the lateral smearing varies with depth as the beamwidth changes, while the axial smearing is the same at all depths.

Also note that the lateral smearing is significantly worse than the axial smearing. Indeed, as a generalisation lateral resolution is worse than axial resolution by at least a factor of three.

This highlights an important practical point:

> *The clearest images of structures (and therefore the best measurements) will be obtained when the structures are perpendicular to the beam direction, i.e. when they are scanned at perpendicular incidence.*

As discussed in chapter 6 the image of the structure will then be degraded only by the axial resolution and it will not be affected by lateral resolution.

Clearly spatial resolution is a significant limitation of ultrasound, particularly when relatively low frequencies must be used to achieve sufficient depth of penetration.

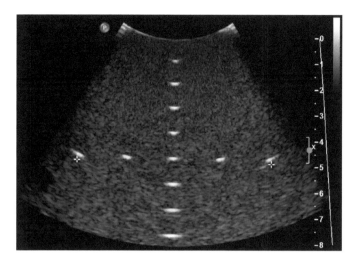

Figure 10.3 Scan of an ultrasound tissue mimicking phantom showing the smearing of a series of regularly spaced point targets.

Contrast resolution

An important question often asked in ultrasound is whether there are areas of abnormal tissue (such as metastases) in an otherwise homogeneous region (such as the liver or thyroid).

This requires the user to be able recognise the abnormal tissues in the image, which means they must differ from the surrounding tissues in some way.

They may have higher or lower attenuation, in which case shadowing or enhancement may be evident. They may differ structurally.

Often, however, the abnormal tissues will be identified because they have higher or lower echogenicity (i.e. they will be brighter or darker in the image) than the surrounding tissues.

At times this difference in echogenicity may be quite small.

Image quality then becomes very important, since subtle differences in echogenicity are less likely to be detected in poor quality images.

The term "contrast resolution" is used in ultrasound to describe the user's ability to detect small differences in soft tissue echogenicity.

As discussed in chapter 6, every ultrasound image contains artifacts (beamwidth, slice thickness, sidelobe, reverberation etc.). While the echoes due to artifacts are not generally identifiable unless they fall into an area which is otherwise echo-free, they still degrade the image.

You may remember the suggestion that it can be useful to think of there being an ideal ultrasound image which is then degraded by the presence of artifacts. The more it is degraded the worse the image quality will be.

In particular, it is clear that the presence of artifacts will worsen contrast resolution. The more spurious echoes there are due to artifacts the worse the contrast resolution will be.

For this reason new modes of operation which reduce artifacts (e.g. harmonic imaging and spatial compound imaging) have become widely used. These will be described in chapter 12.

Are there other factors that affect contrast resolution? Yes. The presence of speckle in soft tissue areas reduces our ability to observe small differences in echogenicity and therefore worsens contrast resolution.

Several techniques have been introduced to reduce speckle, including the use of persistence (discussed below in the context of temporal resolution), spatial compound imaging and image manipulation (see Chapter 12).

In addition, the machine's settings must be optimised for each application, particularly the TGC, gain, dynamic range and ultrasound frequency. Incorrect setting of these controls can degrade contrast resolution.

Temporal resolution

The remaining performance measure is related to movement. The machine's ability to satisfactorily image moving structures is termed its temporal resolution.

In the case of the heart, movement of the heart walls and valve leaflets is integral to its function and we have already discussed the use of M-mode ultrasound to get detailed information regarding these dynamics. 2D ultrasound can also be very useful in this assessment, since areas of abnormal movement may be more easily recognised in a 2D image than in M-mode.

Many other anatomic areas are also subject to movement. Arteries pulsate, and this movement can be transferred to surrounding tissues, making them move too. Abdominal organs move (sometimes quite vigorously) as a result of the patient's breathing.

Clearly the ultrasound machine must have an adequate frame rate to capture and display moving tissues properly.

There is another reason why the frame rate is important.

Often the probe is moved quite quickly over the patient's skin. An inadequate frame rate will cause jerkiness and/or blurring of the image as the probe is moved.

With the introduction of operating modes that use more than one transmit pulse for each line of sight (e.g. colour Doppler, compound imaging, harmonics), frame rates became unacceptably low in some applications.

A solution was found in the form of multiple beamforming. As shown in Figure 10.4, a relatively broad transmit beam is used and several closely spaced receive beams can then receive echoes *simultaneously*.

While this makes the machine's processing more complex, the benefit is that the frame rate is increased in proportion to the number of receive beams. If four simultaneous beams are used as shown in the diagram, the frame rate will increase by a factor of four.

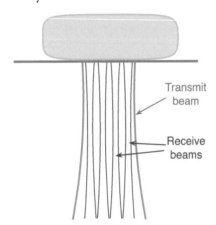

Figure 10.4 Multiple beamforming. A pulse is transmitted down a relatively broad transmit beam. Four closely spaced receive beams gather the returning echoes from this pulse simultaneously. Thus a single transmit pulse has provided echo information for four lines of sight in the image.

In earlier chapters we saw that a number of factors affect the frame rate:

- The PRF, which in turn is limited by the depth of penetration (P).
- The number of lines of sight in each image (L). This is determined primarily by the equipment's designers. However, there may be a control that allows the user to increase line density to emphasise spatial resolution at the expense of frame rate or to decrease line density to achieve higher frame rate at the expense of spatial resolution.
- The number of transmit pulses required for each line of sight (E). For normal imaging this is 1;

for pulse inversion harmonic imaging it is 2; for multiple focus imaging (see Chapter 4) it is equal to the number of foci used; for spatial compound imaging it is equal to the number of images that are combined to produce each displayed image (up to 9, possibly even more).

We know that the relationship between the maximum allowable PRF and the depth of penetration P is:

$$\text{maximum } PRF = \frac{c}{2P}$$

We can see that the number of transmit pulses required for each image (N) is:

$$N = \frac{L \times E}{M}$$

where M is the number of simultaneous beams formed. The maximum possible frame rate will be:

$$FR = \frac{PRF}{N}$$

We can assume that the machine will operate at the maximum possible PRF consistent with the penetration depth.

Substituting for N and PRF therefore, we get:

$$FR = \left(\frac{c}{2P}\right) \div \left(\frac{L \times E}{M}\right)$$
$$= \frac{c \times M}{2 \times P \times L \times E}$$

This can be rewritten as:

$$FR \times P \times L \times E = M \times \frac{c}{2}$$

If we express the frame rate in Hz and the depth of penetration in cm then we can substitute the known value of the propagation speed in cm/sec.

This gives us:

$$FR \times P \times L \times E = M \times 77,000 \text{ cm/sec}$$

This equation summarises how the speed of sound in tissue limits the imaging frame rate. It also shows how frame rate is affected by the depth of penetration (P), the image line density (L), the number of pulses required for each line of sight in the image (E) and the number of beams produced simultaneously using multiple beamforming (M).

Parameter	↑ FR	↓ FR
P	↓	↑
L	↓	↑
E	↓	↑
M	↑	↓

Table 10.1 Table showing the effect of various machine parameters on the frame rate. The centre column shows how each parameter would need to change to achieve an increase in frame rate. The right column shows how they would need to change to decrease the frame rate.

Are there other factors that affect temporal resolution? Yes, the use of persistence. As explained in chapter 5, this function is commonly used because it reduces speckle and therefore improves image quality (particularly contrast resolution).

However, since this is achieved by combining the most recently acquired image with one or more previous images it will clearly increase the blurring of moving structures in the image. For this reason persistence should not be used when temporal resolution must be maximised.

Unfortunately in some machines the frame rate readout can be misleading because it indicates the number of *individual images created within the machine per second* rather than the number of *complete images displayed per second.*

Clearly this will be misleading in any mode of operation where the displayed image is a composite of several individual images.

Examples of this include multiple focus, persistence and spatial compound imaging (described in detail in chapter 12).

Consider a machine operating in spatial compounding mode using a total of 9 different beam steering directions to create each image. Suppose that the *indicated* frame rate is 45 Hz (i.e. 45 images per second), but that it refers to the *number of individual images* acquired per second. Given that each compound image displayed is obtained by combining 9 images, the real rate frame rate will be just (45 ÷ 9) = 5 frames per second.

The temporal resolution will therefore be substantially worse than the user might think if they judged it solely by the *indicated* frame rate of 45 Hz.

Table 10.2 Practical actions that can be taken to improve the various performance parameters.

Type of resolution	Action to improve resolution	Potential drawback
Axial	Increase probe frequency if possible	Reduced sensitivity/penetration
	Use a higher frequency probe	Reduced sensitivity/penetration
	Consider reducing output power	Reduced sensitivity/penetration
	Consider reducing overall gain	Reduced sensitivity/penetration
Lateral	Focus at structure of interest	
	Use multiple focal zones	Reduced temporal resolution
	Use Tissue Harmonic Imaging	May degrade axial resolution
	Consider reducing output power	Reduced sensitivity/penetration
	Consider reducing overall gain	Reduced sensitivity/penetration
	Turn compound imaging off	Increased speckle, worse contrast resolution
Contrast	Increase frequency	Reduced sensitivity/penetration
	Find more homogeneous acoustic window	
	Use Tissue Harmonic Imaging	May degrade axial resolution
	Use compound imaging	Reduced temporal resolution
Temporal	Reduce depth	Reduced field of view
	Reduce sector width	Reduced visible field of view
	Turn off pulse inversion harmonics	Degraded contrast resolution
	Turn off compound imaging	Increased speckle, worse contrast resolution
	Reduce persistence	Increased speckle
	Reduce line density	Degraded lateral resolution
	Reduce number of focal zones	Degraded lateral resolution away from focus

Summary

A number of factors must be considered in assessing ultrasound image quality. The major factors are spatial resolution (both axial and lateral), contrast resolution and temporal resolution.

Spatial resolution is maximised by using as high an ultrasound frequency as possible. Contrast resolution is maximised by reducing image artifacts as much as possible. Temporal resolution is maximised by setting the machine's controls to achieve a high frame rate and minimising the use of the persistence function.

Table 10.2 (see the previous page) summarises a number of practical steps that the user can take for improved imaging.

Assessing equipment performance

So far in this chapter we have been looking at how to think objectively about ultrasound image quality. Now we will consider how the performance of an ultrasound machine can be tested objectively.

Who needs to do this? In the past regular testing was regarded as a necessary part of running a responsible ultrasound practice. However modern machines are far more stable and reliable. Their internal performance is monitored automatically and this information is checked whenever the machine is maintained. Other problems, such as a damaged probe or a malfunctioning display, tend to be obvious and can generally be detected by the user.

Most machines are covered by a maintenance contract. It seems reasonable to rely on the periodic maintenance calls to detect problems. Obviously if you suspect a problem you should arrange a service call as soon as practicable.

Imaging performance

In this section we will briefly review the methods used to test imaging performance. In the following section we will do the same for Doppler performance testing.

How can the imaging performance of a machine be tested? Clearly a test object with known properties must be scanned using standardised settings on the machine.

"Tissue-mimicking ultrasound phantoms" have been developed for this purpose. They are available from a number of manufacturers.

These phantoms are generally made of a gel material with various additives so that the material matches the propagation speed, attenuation and scattering of typical soft tissue. The gel is contained in a plastic box with a soft rubber or plastic membrane on the top through which it is scanned.

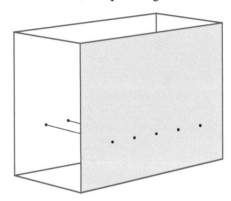

Figure 10.5 Diagram of a typical tissue-mimicking phantom showing a row of five nylon line targets used to test horizontal measurement accuracy.

Some phantoms are made of rubber. They are more robust than gel phantoms, but they cannot achieve the correct propagation speed (1540 m/sec) and this can be a significant disadvantage.

In addition to mimicking soft tissue, phantoms usually provide a series of point targets. These are created by fine nylon lines running across the phantom so they are scanned in cross-section. They are positioned to allow testing of the ultrasound machine's measurement accuracy (both vertical and horizontal) and spatial resolution (both axial and lateral) – see Figure 10.5. Figures 10.6, 10.7 and 10.8 show these tests being carried out on a typical ultrasound phantom.

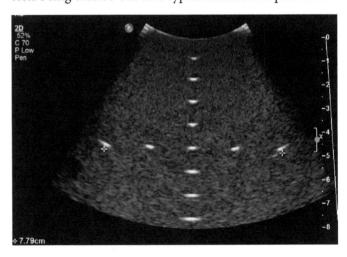

Figure 10.6 Scan of a phantom showing how the accuracy of horizontal measurements is checked. The measured distance between the targets (7.79 cm) differs from the true distance (8.0 cm) by just 2.6% which is within the range of acceptable error.

A number of other features may be incorporated into an imaging phantom. These include:

- contrast resolution targets – cylindrical regions of varying echogenicity, both greater and less than the surrounding material;

- shadowing targets – small, highly attenuating regions;

- division of the phantom into two separate compartments having different attenuation values (e.g. 0.5 dB/cm/MHz and 0.7 dB/cm/MHz) to allow for a wider range of probe frequencies and penetration depths (see Figure 10.9).

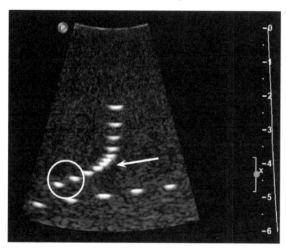

Figure 10.7 (a) Scan of a phantom showing a set of spatial resolution targets. Several of the targets merge together axially and are barely resolved (arrow). Also note that if the targets were all at the same depth only those on the left (circled) would be resolved laterally, the others would merge together in the image.

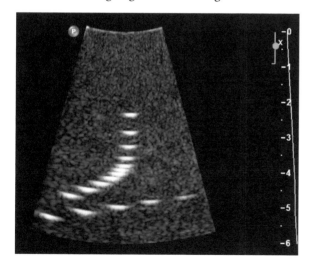

Figure 10.7 (b). With the focus set more superficially the lateral resolution has degraded and none of the targets would be resolved laterally. Notice that the axial resolution is unchanged, since it is not affected by beamwidth.

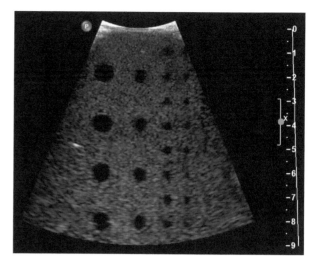

Figure 10.8 (a) Scan of a phantom containing a number of anechoic cylindrical regions with no scatterers. All but the smallest cylinders on the right are resolved and echo-free, though the walls are not sharply defined (particularly away from the focal depth) due to beamwidth effects.

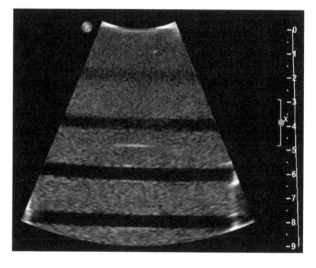

Figure 10.8 (b). When the probe is rotated 90° slice thickness artifact causes echoes from tissues lateral to the cylinders to be displayed within them. The slice thickness must be focussed around 8 cm depth since the cylinder at this depth is most clearly displayed as anechoic.

In addition, specialised phantoms are produced for testing specific functions (e.g. the Doppler phantoms described in the next section) and to simulate specific anatomic regions (e.g. breast, vascular and transvaginal phantoms).

Doppler performance

Designing a phantom for testing Doppler performance is more difficult since it must contain a moving target capable of producing fairly realistic Doppler signals. Two approaches have traditionally been taken, one simplistic and one that is significantly more complex.

The moving string Doppler phantom was introduced earlier. You will recall that a thread is moved at a known speed in a water tank and the scattered signal from the thread provides the Doppler signal (see Figure 10.10).

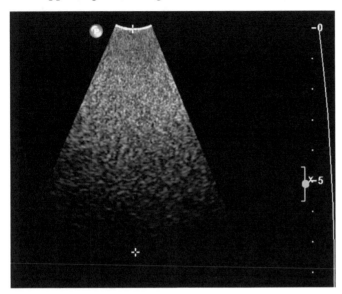

Figure 10.9 The sensitivity of the machine is assessed by noting the approximate depth at which echoes cease to be displayed reliably.

Clearly this ignores many factors – it does not simulate surrounding tissues, or tissue movement, or even the vessel walls. Neither is the target a fluid. Thus it is far from realistic, but it does have the advantage that it provides a moving target with an accurately known velocity.

If a more complete simulation is required then a flow phantom can be used (see Figure 10.11). While it does simulate surrounding tissues and vessel walls, this phantom can have practical difficulties.

The scatterers in the fluid tend to clump, and it can be difficult to avoid the presence of microbubbles within the fluid, which are very strong scatterers.

Furthermore, while the flow rate may be known the velocity profile is unlikely to be parabolic and so the velocity is not known with precision.

Summary

Tissue mimicking and Doppler phantoms can be used to assess equipment performance in a semi-realistic way. Most ultrasound users will not need to use them, since modern ultrasound machines are reliable and unlikely to lose calibration. However, ultrasound machines should be maintained and checked for faults regularly by experienced technicians.

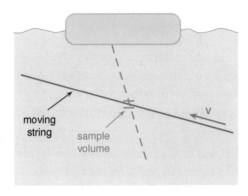

Figure 10.10. In a moving string phantom a precision motor drives a thread around a set of pulley wheels in a water tank. The Doppler signal is acquired from the ultrasound scattered by the thread.

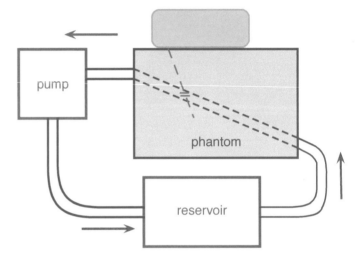

Figure 10.11. In a flow phantom a fluid containing scatterers simulates blood. It is pumped around a loop, passing through a tube embedded in a tissue-mimicking phantom. The tube is generally angled to allow a suitable Doppler angle to be obtained and also to allow Doppler signals to be obtained at different depths.

Suggested activities

1. While scanning, reduce the frame rate (e.g. by using multiple focal depths). Look for any effects on the image such as jerkiness when imaging moving tissues or moving the probe quickly.

2. Look for the effects of lateral and axial resolution. Image a linear structure at perpendicular incidence and then at an angle significantly different from 90°. Note any differences in its appearance.

3. Experiment with persistence and spatial compound scanning (if available on your machine) and note any changes in the speckle seen in relatively uniform soft tissue regions.

Chapter 11

Bioeffects and safety

Is ultrasound safe?

Diagnostic ultrasound is generally considered safe. It does not use ionising radiation like X-rays and it is relatively noninvasive.

Indeed, most policies and statements on the safety of ultrasound by professional organisations include phrases like the following: *"Diagnostic ultrasound has been widely used in clinical medicine for many years with no proven deleterious effects."* (World Federation for Ultrasound in Medicine and Biology Clinical Safety Statement for Diagnostic Ultrasound, accessed from the WFUMB website January 2012).

Nevertheless, the early history of X-rays shows that they too were initially thought to be completely safe. However, it was later found that they can cause cancer which may appear long after the patient's exposure to X-rays.

While ultrasound is very different to X-rays, it is clear that we should use ultrasound with care.

After all, ultrasound is only useful for imaging because it interacts physically with the patient's tissues, exerting mechanical forces on them and heating them. If it passed through the tissues without interacting with them, there would be no echoes and no images.

Moreover, these interactions are sufficiently strong that they can be used therapeutically, for example to heat tissues in physiotherapy and to destroy renal and gall stones in a process called "lithotripsy".

It is possible, though unlikely, that in the future diagnostic ultrasound will be found to have subtle long-term harmful effects due to mechanisms that we have not yet discovered.

Thus we must recognise that:

> *It cannot be proved that ultrasound is completely safe.*

We therefore have an obligation to use it responsibly and only when its use can be justified.

How can we decide whether the use of ultrasound in a specific situation is justified? The answer lies in *the balance between risk and benefit*. Do the expected benefits of the ultrasound examination justify the theoretical risk that it may harm the patient?

The medical literature and clinical experience can provide guidance regarding the expected benefits. We therefore need look at the possible risks. How can they be assessed?

Ideally the safety of ultrasound would be addressed in the same way as a new drug. A randomised controlled trial would be conducted with a large number of subjects. Some of the subjects would be exposed to diagnostic ultrasound and some (the controls) would not. Large numbers of subjects would be required and they would need to be followed up for many years afterwards to identify any harm that may have been caused by the ultrasound.

Unfortunately the time for such a study has passed, since it would be unethical to withhold ultrasound from a substantial number of patients so they could form the control group. This is particularly true of the application area where the safety of ultrasound is of greatest importance – fetal scanning. The benefits of ultrasound in pregnancy are so well established that it would be unacceptable to withhold ultrasound from a group of pregnant patients in order to find out whether there are subtle harmful effects or not.

Some population studies on the safety of ultrasound were done in the past. However, they are of limited relevance today because modern equipment can produce substantially higher intensities than were used at that time.

The possibility that ultrasound can harm tissue must therefore be assessed in other ways. Research has focussed on:

- understanding the interaction of ultrasound with tissue;
- identifying mechanisms by which ultrasound might cause harm;
- determining what factors affect the risk that harm will occur;

- determining how the intensity and duration of the ultrasound exposure affects the risk, and whether there is an exposure threshold below which it can be considered completely safe;
- finding ways to tell the user what the level of risk is for the specific equipment settings being used at the time.

> *TERMINOLOGY*
> *Bioeffect: a physical or mechanical change caused by exposure to ultrasound.*
> *Biohazard: a harmful or potentially harmful bioeffect.*

Mechanisms

First we need to identify the main mechanisms by which ultrasound might cause harm.

Thermal bioeffects

We saw in the second chapter that as ultrasound passes through the patient's tissues some of its energy is lost, causing attenuation. A large part of this loss is due to *absorption* of ultrasound energy, resulting in heating of the tissues.

Thus we know that diagnostic ultrasound will *always* heat the patient's tissues. We also know that excessive heating of tissues can damage them, and that developing fetal tissues are particularly sensitive to raised temperatures.

Thermal mechanisms are therefore singled out as one of the two major categories of bioeffects and/or biohazards.

For convenience, all other mechanisms are gathered together under the heading "mechanical bioeffects".

They will be discussed in the next section.

What determines the amount by which tissues will be heated? Clearly the intensity of the ultrasound exposure is a major factor. As the intensity increases, so will the heating.

The absorption properties of the tissue will also affect heating. Liquids like amniotic fluid absorb virtually no energy while fibrous tissue absorbs much more. Soft tissue such as healthy liver tissue falls in between.

Remember also that the rate of absorption is strongly dependent on the ultrasound frequency. It is far greater at high frequencies than at lower frequencies, and so high frequency probes can be expected to cause more heating.

Another important consideration is whether the beam is scanning through the tissues (as it is in grey scale and colour Doppler imaging) or whether it is stationary (as it is in Pulsed and CW Doppler and M-mode). The more the ultrasound energy is concentrated in a small volume of tissue the greater the heating of that tissue will be.

As mentioned in the Doppler chapter, pulsed Doppler is a particular concern because the beam is kept stationary. In addition, the transmit power used for pulsed Doppler is higher than for grey scale imaging to compensate for the poor scattering properties of blood. Thus:

> *Pulsed Doppler is the mode of operation most likely to cause substantial temperature increases in the patient's tissues.*

Why is CW Doppler less of a concern? There are two reasons.

First, the fact that the transmitted signal is continuous rather than pulsed means that its amplitude is very low compared with pulsed Doppler.

Secondly, CW Doppler uses the simplest possible processing to detect the Doppler signal and so it is very efficient.

This means that it requires less transmit power to achieve a certain level of signal in CW Doppler than it does in pulsed Doppler.

There is yet another factor that must be considered. As the tissues in a given location heat up, some of the heat is transferred to adjacent tissues by conduction. This will spread the heat through a larger volume of tissue, reducing the temperature rise. (Think of a saucepan on a stove. The heat is applied to the bottom of the pan but the entire saucepan becomes hot through conduction of the heat.)

Blood flow is a major contributor to this effect, since the blood will carry away some of the excess heat, distributing it throughout the body. (Think how the cooling system and radiator in a car keep the engine from overheating.) Thus well perfused tissues will heat up considerably less than poorly perfused tissues.

Interfaces between soft tissue and bone are a particular concern. A large part of the ultrasound energy is reflected at these interfaces. The remainder is transmitted into the bone, undergoing a process known as "mode conversion" as it moves from soft tissue to bone. This causes substantial localised heating at the soft tissue/bone interface.

What is an acceptable temperature increase? Naturally the answer varies depending on the nature of the tissues.

Fetal tissues are particularly sensitive to heating.

It is widely agreed that a temperature increase of up to 1.5°C *above normal body temperature* can be tolerated by a fetus without harm, even if the raised temperature is sustained for a considerable time. On the other hand, a temperature increase of 4.0°C or more is regarded as dangerous for the fetus, even for a short time, and should be avoided.

Note that the above statement talks about the amount by which the temperature increases "above normal body temperature" (37°C). Consider again the 1.5°C temperature increase mentioned above. This means that for the fetus the maximum acceptable sustained tissue temperature is (37°C + 1.5°C) = 38.5°C.

If a patient has a fever, the permissible amount of heating will clearly be reduced. A body temperature of 37.5°C, for example, would mean that only a 1.0°C temperature increase would be acceptable for a sustained period.

How can the likely temperature rise in a given scanning situation be determined?

The machine calculates the likely rise on the basis of the exposure factors (which it knows), namely the:

- transmit power;
- frequency;
- focal depth;
- scanning mode.

It will also take account of the clinical application area (fetal, peripheral vascular, upper abdominal etc) since this will affect the types of tissue likely to be involved.

A considerable number of assumptions must be made in this calculation, including:

- how much the transmitted ultrasound will be attenuated as it travels through the tissues to the depth where the heating is greatest;
- the absorption properties of the tissues;
- the heat conduction properties of the tissues;
- the amount of blood flow through the tissues.

While these assumptions are usually reasonably accurate, they will not always be correct. For example, the beam path may be more or less attenuating than would normally be expected.

If the user knows that one or more of the assumptions made by the machine in estimating the temperature increase is likely to be wrong then they must factor this into their interpretation of the machine's estimate of the temperature rise.

The estimated temperature increase is displayed by the machine as the "Thermal Index" (or TI).

While the formal definition of the TI is more complex, it is essentially a measure of the likely maximum temperature rise in the patient's tissues in °C. For example, a TI of 0.8 means that the likely temperature rise due to the ultrasound exposure will be 0.8°C.

For situations where the majority of the tissues are soft tissue, the index is referred to as the "soft tissue" Thermal Index (TIs or TIS).

Where bones are present in the region of interest (e.g. the fetal skeleton in second and third trimester pregnancies) the extra heating that occurs at the soft tissue/bone interface must be taken into account. The relevant index is then the "bone" Thermal Index (TIb or TIB).

Bone may also lie *between* the probe and the region of interest. In cerebral examinations, for example, the probe is placed in close proximity to the patient's skull. This situation is catered for by using the "cranial" Thermal Index (TIc or TIC).

Note that some machines will not display the Thermal Index unless its value is greater than 1.0. You may even encounter a machine which does not display the Thermal Index at all. This is likely to indicate that its manufacturers have instead complied with regulatory safety requirements by limiting its ultrasound output to levels that are considered completely safe. This is discussed in more detail later in this chapter.

In summary therefore, ultrasound will always cause some degree of heating in the patient's tissues. The maximum temperature increase is estimated continuously by the machine as you scan and it is generally displayed on the screen in the form of the Thermal Index. This provides guidance as to whether the amount of heating is within safe limits or whether it should be of concern. At times additional factors need to be taken into account, e.g. if the patient has a fever.

Mechanical bioeffects

A number of non-thermal effects have been observed.

The most important is "cavitation". This term is used to describe the behaviour of gas bubbles when they are exposed to ultrasound. Cavitation is important because (a) gas bubbles are regularly found in areas such as the lungs and gastrointestinal tract and (b) cavitation can be extremely harmful.

As we saw in an earlier chapter, ultrasound causes oscillating pressures in the tissues as it passes through them.

How do these pressure variations affect any gas bubbles that are present in the tissues? As the pressure increases, the bubbles are compressed and so they reduce in size. As the pressure decreases they expand. In some situations this oscillation of the bubbles is stable. This is known as "non-inertial" cavitation. At other times, however, the bubbles will implode (i.e. collapse very rapidly), generating a shock wave and exposing the tissues in the immediate area to high stresses. This "inertial" cavitation is potentially very damaging.

What are the main factors affecting the risk of cavitation? First, cavitation can only occur when gas bubbles are present in the tissues. Second, the risk of cavitation increases as the ultrasound intensity increases, as we would expect. Third, as shown by the equation below, the risk of cavitation is greatest at low frequencies, decreasing as the ultrasound frequency increases.

By its nature, cavitation cannot be quantified in the same way as the temperature increase. Instead the "Mechanical Index" (MI) has been defined as follows:

$$MI = \frac{P_r}{\sqrt{f}}$$

P_r is the peak rarefaction pressure (expressed in Pascals), i.e. the greatest negative pressure (see Figure 11.1) and f is the ultrasound frequency (expressed in MHz).

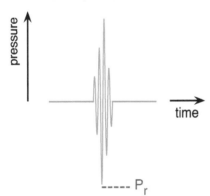

Figure 11.1 A typical transmit pulse showing the definition of the peak rarefaction pressure P_r.

As with the Thermal Index, the Mechanical Index is displayed by the ultrasound machine to allow the user to decide whether the current machine settings can be considered as safe or whether there is some risk to the patient (see Figure 11.2).

The interpretation of the MI is less straightforward than the interpretation of the TI, since it does not relate directly to a physical quantity like heat.

Instead the MI should be seen as a number designed to indicate the risk of cavitation. The maximum acceptable value for the MI is generally agreed to be 1.9.

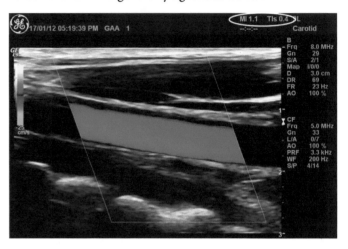

Figure 11.2 Colour Doppler image with the MI and TIs displayed (circled).

Apart from cavitation, have any other non-thermal bioeffects been identified? Yes, "radiation force" has been shown to be capable of causing bioeffects. This term refers to the force exerted on any object that reflects or absorbs ultrasound. Indeed, there are devices which use radiation force to measure the output power of ultrasound systems (see Figure 11.3).

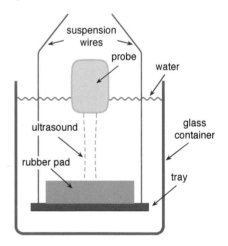

Figure 11.3 A radiation force system used to measure the output power of an ultrasound probe. The force generated on the rubber pad is directly proportional to the transmitted ultrasound power level. The pad is resting on a tray suspended from a weighing scale which measures the force. This technique can provide a very accurate measure of the output power.

A common result of ultrasound radiation force is movement of liquids such as blood which contain particles that reflect or absorb ultrasound. In general this "streaming" is considered harmless at diagnostic intensity levels.

More importantly, however, it is believed that radiation force is likely to be the explanation for the bleeding that has been observed in the capillaries of lung tissue exposed (in research settings) to ultrasound at moderately high intensities.

Researchers have suggested that the incident ultrasound generates sufficient force when it reflects from gas in the alveoli to damage adjacent tissues and cause some of the capillaries to bleed.

The Mechanical Index is believed to be a reasonable guide to the likelihood of harm due to radiation force effects (and other non-thermal effects that may exist), as well as being an indication of the likelihood of cavitation.

In summary, a number of mechanical (i.e. non-thermal) bioeffects have been identified. Of greatest concern is cavitation, which can occur in the presence of gas bubbles and can cause localised tissue damage. Radiation force is also of concern given the likelihood that it is the cause of capillary bleeding seen in lungs exposed to moderately high exposure. The Mechanical Index is designed to indicate the risk of harmful effects from non-thermal mechanisms. The accepted safe limit for the MI is 1.9.

Suggested activities

1. As you are scanning, note the displayed Thermal Index and Mechanical Index values.

2. See whether the displayed TI type (i.e. TIs, TIb or TIc) changes depending on the clinical application area selected.

3. Compare the TI and MI values in different operating modes (grey scale imaging, colour Doppler, pulsed Doppler etc).

4. Change some of the machine's parameters (e.g. the transmit power and frequency, depth of focus, pulsed Doppler velocity scale, colour Doppler box width etc). Note any changes in the TI and MI. Are these changes consistent with what you expected?

Characterising ultrasound exposure

An earlier chapter introduced the concepts of energy, power and intensity (see Table 11.1). Since we want a measure of *tissue exposure*, intensity is the most useful parameter, since it specifies how much energy passes through a given volume of tissue each second (see Figure 11.4).

Quantity	Definition	Units
energy	total "work" done	Joules
power	energy per second	Watts
intensity	power per square centimetre	W/cm²

Table 11.1 Definitions of the parameters used to measure ultrasound exposure.

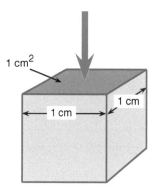

Figure 11.4 The term "intensity" specifies the amount of ultrasound energy (blue arrow) passing through one square centimetre of tissue.

When we start to look at just how to calculate the intensity, however, we quickly realise that there are complicating factors that must be taken into account. The transducer does not transmit continuously (except in CW Doppler). Instead it transmits short pulses of ultrasound with substantial intervals between them to allow echoes to be received. We refer to this as the *temporal* variation of the ultrasound exposure (see Figure 11.5).

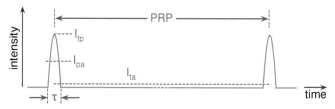

Figure 11.5 Temporal variation of the transmitted ultrasound. PRP is the pulse repetition period (i.e. the time from one transmit pulse to the next), τ is the transmit pulse duration and I_{tp}, I_{pa} and I_{ta} are the temporal peak, pulse average and temporal average intensities respectively.

A useful concept is the duty factor (sometimes called the "duty cycle"). This is simply the fraction of time for which the transducer is transmitting, that is:

$$DF = \frac{\tau}{PRP}$$

where DF is the duty factor, τ is the duration of the transmit pulse and PRP is the pulse repetition period (you may remember that the PRP is simply equal to (1/PRF)).

Typical values for the duty factor in grey scale imaging range from 0.1% to 1%. They are somewhat higher for pulsed Doppler due to the longer transmit pulse duration used in Doppler.

The pulse average intensity I_{pa} is simply the intensity averaged over the transmit pulse duration. It can therefore be written as:

$$I_{pa} = \frac{P_p}{\tau}$$

where P_p is the energy per square centimetre contained in one transmit pulse and τ is the pulse duration.

As Figure 11.5 shows, the pulse average intensity is somewhat lower than the temporal peak intensity I_{tp}.

The temporal average intensity I_{ta} is calculated by averaging the intensity over the entire pulse repetition period PRP. It can therefore be written as:

$$I_{ta} = \frac{P_p}{PRP}$$

Combining these equations we can see that there is a simple relationship between the temporal average and pulse average intensity values:

$$\frac{I_{ta}}{I_{pa}} = \left(\frac{P_p}{PRP}\right) \div \left(\frac{P_p}{\tau}\right)$$
$$= \left(\frac{P_p}{PRP}\right) \times \left(\frac{\tau}{P_p}\right)$$
$$= \frac{\tau}{PRP}$$
$$= DF$$

and therefore:

$$I_{ta} = I_{pa} \times DF$$

Since the duty factor is typically 0.1% - 1.0%, we can see that the temporal average intensity will be very much smaller than the pulse average and temporal peak intensities.

The ultrasound intensity also varies both with depth and across the beam at any given depth. This is the *spatial* variation of the ultrasound exposure (see Figure 11.6).

Looking at Figure 11.6 we can see that the maximum intensity (the spatial peak intensity I_{sp}) will be found at the focal depth and on the central axis of the beam. In fact this is not strictly true. Once we take attenuation of the ultrasound into account it is clear that the intensity values will decrease progressively with depth. As a result, the spatial peak value will occur on the beam axis but somewhat closer to the probe than the actual focal point.

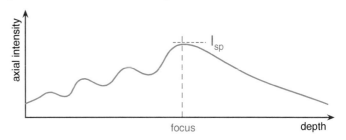

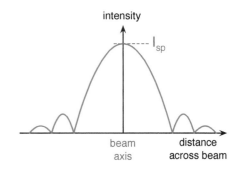

Figure 11.6 Spatial variation of the intensity: (Top) variation along the beam's axis with depth and (bottom) variation across the beam at a given depth.

Yet another intensity value has been defined. This is the spatial average intensity I_{sa}, defined as the transmit intensity averaged over the face of the transducer.

Since the focussed beamwidth is generally substantially narrower than the transducer face, the intensity within the tissues will be considerably higher than the spatial average intensity, making it a relatively meaningless parameter. Unfortunately, however, it is the easiest intensity value to measure and so it is often quoted in manufacturers' specifications and publications.

Thus we have seen that there are a number of intensity values available. These are summarised in Table 11.2.

Intensity	Symbol	Relative Magnitude
spatial peak temporal peak	I_{sptp}	1000
spatial peak pulse average	I_{sppa}	500
spatial average temporal peak	I_{satp}	100
spatial peak temporal average	I_{spta}	1
spatial average temporal average	I_{sata}	0.1

Table 11.2 Definitions of the various measures of intensity and rough approximations of their relative magnitudes.

The choice of which to use depends on the circumstances. Heating is a relatively slow phenomenon, since the temperature increase occurs over a period of many seconds, so the temporal average intensity will be the relevant parameter. Heat spreads out through the tissues and so the spatial average is also the relevant parameter. Thus the spatial average temporal average intensity I_{sata} is most relevant to heating.

In contrast, highly localised phenomena are likely to be determined by the instantaneous maximum local exposure, in which case the spatial peak and temporal peak intensity I_{sptp} is more relevant.

Government regulation

Who sets the standards for ultrasound equipment manufacturers? In principle, different regulations apply in different parts of the world. However, in practice the ultrasound equipment market has become so globalised that the great majority of manufacturers comply with the regulations prescribed by the Food and Drug Administration (FDA) in the United States. We will therefore focus in this section on the regulation of ultrasound equipment output levels in the United States.

In its early years, ultrasound equipment was not officially regulated on the grounds that it was a non-ionising form of radiation and believed to be totally safe at clinical levels of exposure. By 1976, however, the use of ultrasound was growing rapidly and the FDA was given responsibility for regulating equipment output levels in the United States.

Relatively little was known at that time regarding the mechanisms of ultrasound bioeffects and so the FDA took a pragmatic approach.

Since there had been no substantiated reports of harm to patients due to ultrasound exposure, it was felt that the output levels used in equipment up to that time should be regarded as safe.

A survey was therefore conducted to determine the upper limits of the exposure levels produced by equipment used up to 1976 in various categories of application (peripheral vascular, cardiac, ophthalmic, fetal and other).

These "pre-1976" exposure limits became the mandated upper limits for equipment manufactured after 1976.

Further research on bioeffects and safety was encouraged in the hope that it could provide the basis for a more scientific approach to be taken to regulation. By the early 1990s it was felt that the two main mechanisms – thermal and cavitation – were sufficiently understood to warrant a change in the FDA's approach to regulation.

The on-screen display of the Thermal and Mechanical Indices was therefore introduced.

Since that time the FDA has offered manufacturers the choice between two "tracks" for obtaining approval of their equipment.

"Track 1" retains the pre-1976 approach (with minor modifications). The output limits for Track 1 are shown in Table 11.3. Note that they are "derated" assuming a (rather conservative) attenuation value of 0.3 dB/cm/MHz.

Use	$I_{spta.3}$ (mW/cm²)	$I_{sppa.3}$ (mW/cm²)	MI
peripheral vascular	720	190	1.9
cardiac	430	190	1.9
fetal & "other"	94	190	1.9
ophthalmic	17	28	0.23

Table 11.3 Output limits specified by the FDA under Track 1. The values are "derated" assuming an attenuation value of 0.3 dB/cm/MHz. Manufacturers must meet the I_{spta} limit and either the MI limit or the I_{sppa} limit. ["Other" means abdominal, intraoperative, paediatric, small parts, neonatal cephalic and adult cephalic applications.]

"Track 3" requires that the TI and MI be displayed on the machine whenever the probe-machine combination is capable of producing a value for either index greater than 1.0.

In addition, the FDA has imposed global upper limits on the (derated) value of specific output parameters as follows:

$I_{spta} < 720$ mW/cm^2 and

$MI < 1.9$ or

$I_{sppa} < 190$ W/cm^2

For ophthalmic applications substantially lower global limits have been set:

$TI < 1$ and

$I_{spta} < 50$ mW/cm^2 and

$MI < 0.3$

Importantly, the introduction of Track 3 has allowed manufacturers to significantly increase the output power levels that their equipment is capable of producing. This has been welcomed by most users since it has made it easier to achieve adequate penetration in "difficult" patients and has made it possible to extend the use of higher frequency probes.

More importantly, Track 3 represents a dramatic shift in philosophy. The Track 1 approach was based on the idea that manufacturers would be required to produce machines that were totally safe.

Track 3 allows machines to be able to produce higher outputs on the grounds that it also provides the user with the means to monitor the risk level for the patient and to assess whether the balance between risk and benefit is appropriate. In recognition of this, the FDA has stipulated that under Track 3 manufacturers must provide end users of their equipment with education on bioeffects, safety, risk-benefit analysis and the ALARA principle (the latter will be discussed in the next section). To repeat this very important point:

> *Modern equipment can produce higher exposure levels in the patient than was permitted in the past. This means it is essential for the user to monitor the TI and MI values that are displayed as they scan, and to understand what they mean.*

Policies and statements

Where else can the user get advice regarding the safety of diagnostic ultrasound? Professional organisations such as the World Federation for Ultrasound in Medicine and Biology (WFUMB), the American Institute of Ultrasound in Medicine (AIUM), the British Medical Ultrasound Society (BMUS) and the Australasian Society for Ultrasound in Medicine (ASUM) publish policy statements and guidelines. These are readily available online and you should read them and be familiar with their recommendations.

In summary, these policies generally make the following points:

- ultrasound has been used for decades and has proved highly valuable;
- it has an excellent safety record, with no confirmed reports of patients being harmed by diagnostic exposure levels;
- nevertheless it is impossible to prove that ultrasound is totally safe; there may be subtle harmful effects that have not yet been identified, especially since modern equipment can produce higher exposure levels than those used historically;
- it is therefore essential that ultrasound is used responsibly and only when the benefit justifies any possible risk there may be to the patient;
- the TI and MI give the user guidance as to the level of risk that the patient is being exposed to;
- ultrasound should not be used in situations where there is no expected medical benefit;
- ultrasound should therefore only be used when medically indicated, or for teaching and research;
- thus the use of ultrasound to produce "keepsake" images of the fetus is inappropriate if it prolongs the examination;
- the guiding principle when using ultrasound should be the ALARA principle.

What is the ALARA principle? It says:

> *The exposure of the patient to ultrasound should be As Low As Reasonably Achievable (ALARA) consistent with obtaining the necessary clinical information.*

This applies to the exposure levels (as indicated by the TI and MI) and the duration of the exposure.

Thus you should be aware of the TI and MI values as you scan and you should not prolong the patient exposure to ultrasound unnecessarily.

Note the emphasis on "reasonably achievable". You should not become over-concerned about safety to the point of compromising the clinical value of your scan.

For example, the preset output power levels selected by the machine at the start of the examination will normally be well within safe limits. Reducing the transmit power would therefore be unnecessary, time-wasting and could potentially reduce the quality of the clinical information.

On the other hand, you should not continue scanning the patient while you review images, make measurements etc; use the freeze button or lift the probe off the patient.

You should also practise answering the question posed at the start of this chapter "is ultrasound safe?" Patients will almost certainly ask you this from time to time. You need to be truthful, succinct and avoid alarming them.

Are there any other risks associated with the ultrasound exam? Yes, you should always remember that:

> *The greatest potential for harm to the patient in diagnostic ultrasound comes from poor quality ultrasound practice: sub-optimal scans, poor reporting, misdiagnosis etc.*

Summary

Ultrasound is relatively safe, particularly when compared with ionising radiation. However, several mechanisms have been identified by which it can harm tissues (and therefore patients). These are:

- heating
- cavitation
- radiation force

There may well be other mechanisms that have not yet been identified.

Modern ultrasound equipment can produce higher levels of tissue exposure than in the past. It is therefore essential that you to monitor the ultrasound exposure of your patients as you scan. The machine displays the Thermal and Mechanical Indices (TI and MI) to help you do this.

In general the following upper limits should be observed:

> TI < 1.5
>
> MI < 1.9

In some circumstances lower limits should be applied.

Many professional ultrasound societies provide guidance to users regarding safety and bioeffects. Usually this takes the form of statements on safety and guidelines for safe use. These should be followed at all times. The main features of the guidelines are that ultrasound should only be used when medically indicated and the ALARA principle, which specifies that the exposure levels and duration should be as low as reasonably achievable.

You should note that the information in this chapter was correct (to the best of the author's knowledge) at the time of writing. However it is quite likely that it may change as researchers learn more about the mechanisms of interaction of ultrasound with tissue. It is your responsibility as a health professional to remain up to date in your knowledge and practice.

Suggested Activities

1. Locate and download the ultrasound safety policies and guidelines of at least two major professional organisations.

2. Read these and compare their approach. Summarise their practical take-home messages.

Chapter 12

Additional modes and capabilities

Introductory comments

Up to this point we have been dealing with the fundamentals of diagnostic ultrasound technology.

In this chapter you will be introduced to a number of refinements. These have been developed over the years to improve and extend what ultrasound can do and to make it easier to use.

Some of them are still evolving, others are long-established and have become a routine part of the equipment.

The topics to be covered in this chapter are:

- compound scanning
- harmonics
- ultrasound contrast agents
- 3D and 4D ultrasound
- extended field of view
- image optimisation
- image manipulation
- elastography

The length of this list underlines the statement made in the first chapter of this book: "A feature of the industry has been constant technological innovation, with new modes of operation being added on a regular basis."

With the knowledge you have gained from the preceding chapters you should now be able to understand these and other new technologies as they are introduced and evolve.

Compound imaging

Why was compound scanning introduced?

As Figure 12.1 shows, conventional scans (sometimes referred to as "simple" scans to differentiate them from compound scans) usually provide incomplete information regarding tissue boundaries.

As explained in the Reflection section in chapter 2, this is due to the fact that only echoes from surfaces which are close to perpendicular to the beam will return to the transducer. Echoes from surfaces at other angles relative to the beam will be reflected away from the transducer and so they will not be seen in the image.

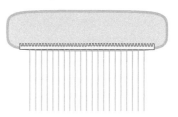

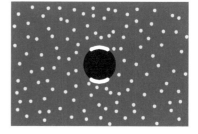

Figure 12.1 This diagram shows how a transverse scan of a blood vessel embedded in soft tissue might look in a conventional (simple) scan. Note that only the top and bottom of the vessel wall are well displayed due to specular reflection. The dots represent speckle from soft tissue scattering.

Compound scanning was introduced to address this limitation. Its principle is shown in Figure 12.2.

While this diagram shows only three images for simplicity, up to nine images may be used in practice, each with a different beam direction. The user is generally able to alter the number of images used by the machine to create the compound image.

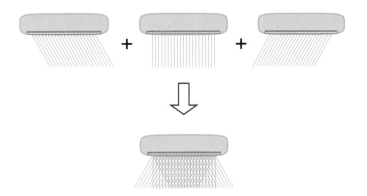

Figure 12.2 In a compound scan several images are formed in rapid succession and combined to form a single "compound" image.

Figure 12.3 shows two important consequences of compound imaging. The first is that curved surfaces (such as the walls of the blood vessel in the diagram) will be more completely displayed in the compound image than they were in the simple scan.

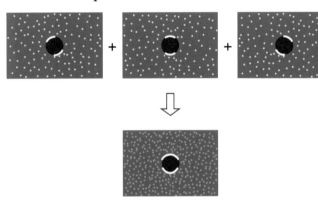

Figure 12.3 Both the echoes from the vessel wall and the speckle from soft tissue will be different in each image. The result is that the compound image will show a more complete image of the vessel wall and the speckle will be smoother.

A second advantage of compound imaging relates to the speckle pattern from soft tissues. The process of combining several different images together leads to a more uniform speckle pattern. It appears smoother to the eye and so it will be less distracting than the coarser speckle found in a conventional (simple) scan.

This is important. Smoothing the speckle improves the user's ability to see subtle variations in the tissues and so it improves the contrast resolution.

Figures 12.4 and 12.5 show two clinical examples of the use of compound scanning.

A third consequence of compound imaging relates to image artifacts.

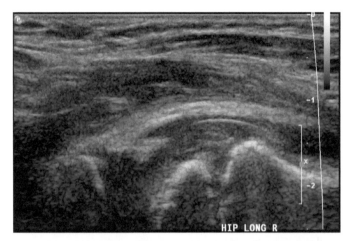

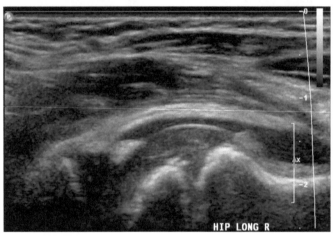

Figure 12.4 A conventional image (top) and a compound image (bottom) of a paediatric hip. In the compound image the tissue speckle is considerably less distracting and the tissue boundaries and fascia are better seen.

As we saw earlier, many artifacts are directed parallel to the beam direction (e.g. shadowing, enhancement, edge shadowing, reverberation, ring-down, comet-tail). This means that their position will be different in each of the images that go to make up the compound image. As Figure 12.6 shows, the result is that they will be far less visible in the compound image than in a simple scan.

A useful way to think of this effect is as follows: each image is made up of a "true" image plus artifactual echoes. When the images are combined to produce the compound image, the "true" image will be the same in each case and so it will be reinforced; the artifacts will be different in each image and so they will be diminished in the compound image. Figure 12.7 is a clinical example showing marked reduction of enhancement due to compound imaging.

Much the same is true of other image artifacts. Beamwidth and sidelobe effects will be also different in each of the individual images and so they too will be reduced in the compound image.

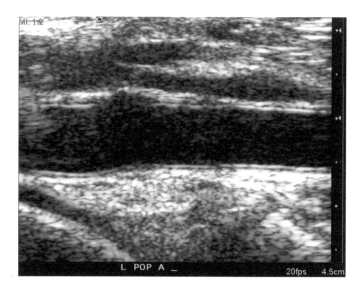

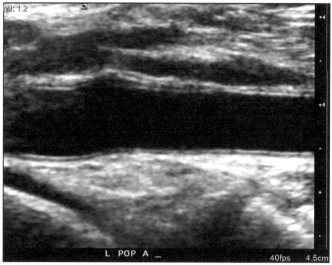

Figure 12.5 A comparison of (top) a simple scan of a popliteal artery and (bottom) the same artery imaged using compound scanning. Again the speckle is substantially smoother and tissue boundaries are better seen in the compound image.

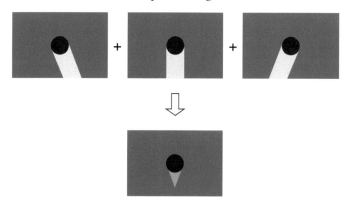

Figure 12.6 This diagram shows enhancement due to a blood vessel. When the three images are combined, the enhancement will be reduced since it is in a different position in each of the individual images.

At this point it may seem that compound imaging has so many advantages that it should be the standard mode of operation. It improves the visualisation of tissue boundaries, reduces distracting speckle and reduces most artifacts.

Unfortunately it has two major disadvantages. Most obviously, the frame rate and temporal resolution are substantially worsened due to the fact that each displayed image requires the acquisition of up to nine standard images. (As mentioned previously, the frame rate displayed on the machine may be misleading since it may show the number of simple scan images acquired each second, rather than the number of compound images.)

Less obvious is the fact that some artifacts (e.g. the enhancement in Figure 12.7) are valuable and their loss or reduction in the compound image may not be desirable. Given these two considerations – the reduced frame rate and loss of useful artifacts – compound imaging is generally regarded as a secondary imaging mode and so it is used selectively.

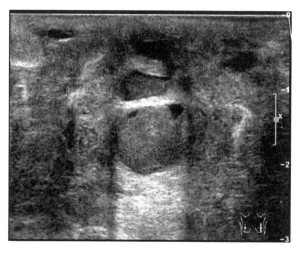

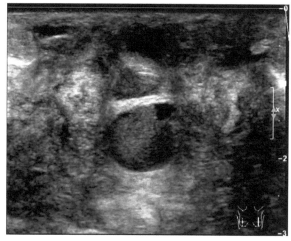

Figure 12.7 A simple scan (top) and a compound scan (bottom) of a breast abscess. The enhancement caused by the abscess is obvious in the simple scan but it is difficult to see in the compound image.

Suggested activities

1. Experiment with compound scanning in several different application areas.

2. Acquire simple and compound scans of the same anatomy and compare them. Note any improvements in the images and any changes in artifacts.

Harmonics

In chapters 2 and 3 you were introduced to the concept of "frequency analysis". It was explained that a single-frequency wave, by definition, is a perfect sine wave which continues for all time.

Any other wave – whether it has a different shape than a perfect sine wave or whether it exists for only a finite time – can be built up by adding together a number of sine waves of different frequencies and amplitudes. This is called "frequency analysis" of the wave.

In particular, chapter 2 showed that a wave with frequency f but with a triangular shape is made up of the sum of sine waves with frequencies of f, 2f, 3f etc (see Figure 12.8).

Thus, frequency analysis of the triangular wave has revealed that it is made up of a "fundamental" component (a sine wave with frequency f), a second harmonic component (a sine wave with frequency 2f), a third harmonic component (a sine wave with frequency 3f), …. etc.

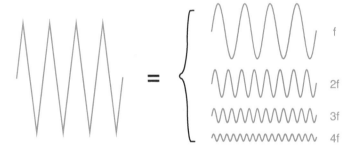

Figure 12.8 A triangular wave is the sum of the fundamental frequency and its harmonics.

In fact it can be shown that *any* repetitive wave that is not a perfect sine wave is the sum of a fundamental component (equal to its repetition frequency) and a series of harmonics.

How is this relevant to ultrasound?

If the echo signal received by the ultrasound machine is "distorted" for any reason then it will no longer be purely sinusoidal and some of its energy will be at harmonic frequencies.

This concept is the basis for both Tissue Harmonic Imaging (THI) and Contrast Harmonics (the use of harmonic imaging with ultrasound contrast agents).

Figure 12.8 relates to a continuous wave. In reality the transmitted signal is generally a short pulse of ultrasound, so we need to know what happens when a pulse is distorted.

In chapter 3 it was explained that frequency analysis of a pulse shows it to be the sum of an infinite number of sine waves over a defined range of frequencies (see Figure 12.9).

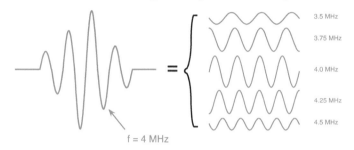

Figure 12.9 (a) A 4 MHz pulse with a duration of 1 μsec is the sum of an infinite number of frequencies ranging from 3.5 MHz to 4.5 MHz.

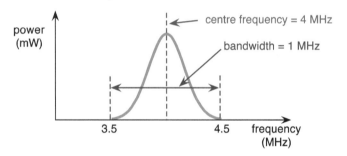

Figure 12.9 (b) A more convenient way to display the frequency content of the pulse is as a frequency spectrum.

When a pulse is distorted, harmonics will be generated, just as with a continuous wave. However *all* the frequencies present in the pulse will be affected and so we find that the entire pulse spectrum is repeated at harmonic intervals, as shown in Figure 12.10.

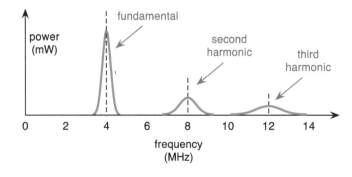

Figure 12.10 When an ultrasound pulse becomes distorted its entire spectrum is repeated at harmonic intervals.

Our main interest is to understand the implications of the above for the echoes received by the ultrasound machine.

Since we know that each echo is a replica of the transmit pulse, it follows that:

> *Echoes will be distorted whenever the transmit pulse is distorted. They will then have a significant component of energy at the second harmonic frequency.*

Tissue Harmonic Imaging (THI)

When and how does the transmit pulse become distorted? As ultrasound passes through tissue it increases and decreases the pressure in the tissue, as described in chapter 2.

If the ultrasound intensity is relatively low then this has little effect on the physical properties of the tissue. However, if the intensity is high then the pressure changes are sufficient to cause significant physical changes. In particular, when the pressure is increased the tissue becomes stiffer, and when the pressure is reduced the tissue becomes more elastic.

What effect does this have on the ultrasound wave?

The most important effect is that as the tissue stiffness increases, so does the ultrasound propagation speed. Conversely, when the tissue becomes more elastic, the propagation speed is reduced (see Figure 12.11).

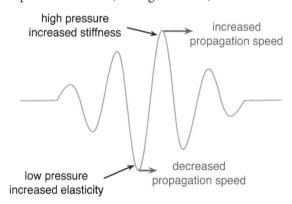

Figure 12.11 When the ultrasound intensity is high the pressure variations that it causes will affect the propagation speed as shown here. The differences in propagation speed will cause progressive distortion of the pulse as it propagates through the tissues.

The consequence of these propagation speed changes is that the peaks will travel slightly more quickly than the troughs, causing the pulse to gradually become distorted as it travels through the tissue (see Figure 12.12).

This looks very similar to what happens when ocean waves approach a beach.

Large waves lose their sinusoidal shape (which they had in the open sea) and they become steeper. Smaller waves and ripples don't do this, they remain essentially unchanged until they hit the shore.

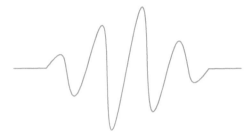

Figure 12.12 Thus, as a high intensity pulse travels through tissue the peaks move to the right and the troughs to the left, causing the waveform shape to "steepen" like an ocean wave that is approaching the shore.

We are now ready to discuss how the machine operates in Tissue Harmonic Imaging (THI) mode. The machine transmits a normal transmit pulse. Due to the mechanism described above, the pulse becomes progressively distorted as it travels into the patient's tissues. Most importantly:

> *The transmitted ultrasound pulse is distorted only in those areas where the intensity is relatively high, i.e. along the central axis of the main beam.*

This means that the echoes coming from these tissues will be distorted, and so they will contain significant energy at the harmonic frequencies. Echoes from other areas will not be distorted and they will have no harmonic energy. Thus, by good fortune we have a situation that allows us to differentiate between echoes coming from the central zone of the main beam and other echoes (see Figure 12.13).

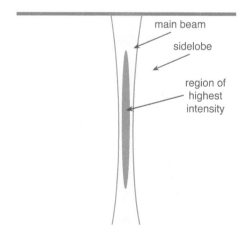

Figure 12.13 The transmit pulse will be distorted as it travels in the high intensity part of the beam (dark blue). In other parts of the main beam and in the sidelobes the intensity is lower and little distortion will occur.

We can exploit this difference in the echoes by making an image that ignores the fundamental frequency and uses *only* the harmonics. We will then see only the echoes coming from the central zone of the beam.

In practice the machine uses just the *second harmonic* to make the image, since the higher harmonics are too low in amplitude and attenuate too quickly to be usable.

For example, if the machine is transmitting at 4 MHz the image will be created using the second harmonic echo information at 8 MHz.

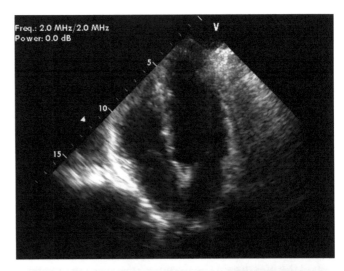

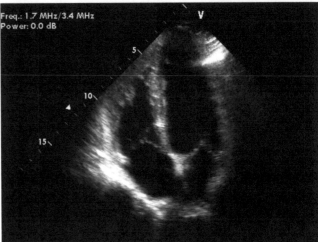

Figure 12.15 Harmonic imaging (bottom) substantially reduces the artifacts often seen within the heart chambers. Many echocardiographers therefore use harmonics as their standard imaging mode.

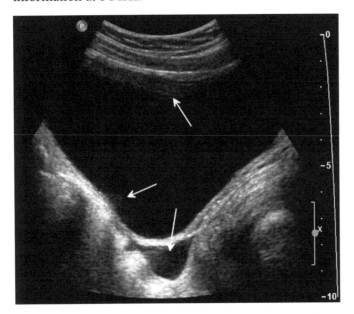

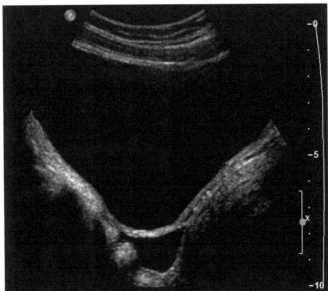

Figure 12.14 A conventional image (top) and a harmonic image (bottom) of the bladder in a paediatric patient. The harmonic image shows a dramatic reduction in reverberation and other artifacts (arrows). Beamwidth effects are also reduced, giving cleaner boundaries between tissue and fluid. However, note the reduced penetration depth.

Tissue Harmonic images are better than conventional images. Why is this? There are two main reasons.

1. As discussed above, harmonic echoes will only come from structures near the axis of the main beam. Since the sidelobes have considerably lower intensity than the main beam, no harmonic echoes should be received from the tissues within the sidelobes. Similarly the outer fringes of the main beam, and of the slice thickness of the beam, have relatively low intensity and so harmonic echoes will not come from these regions either. Thus the image will contain echoes only from the central part of the main beam. Beamwidth, sidelobe and slice thickness artifacts will all be dramatically reduced.

2. As explained above, the transmit pulse gradually becomes distorted as it travels into the patient's tissues. In the first centimetre or two of the tissue it

will therefore be relatively undistorted. This means that echoes from superficial tissues will be relatively weak when imaged using THI. The importance of this is that much of the reverberation seen in images is caused by multiple reflection of the ultrasound within the superficial tissues. Because the transmit pulse is relatively undistorted at this depth, the reverberation echoes contain little energy at the harmonic frequencies. Reverberation artifact is therefore significantly reduced.

Tissue Harmonic Imaging therefore improves image quality by reducing beamwidth, sidelobe, slice thickness and reverberation artifacts. Are there any negatives associated with it? Yes, performance is reduced in two important ways:

1. Being at a higher frequency the second harmonic attenuates far more rapidly than the fundamental, so the depth of penetration is significantly reduced.

2. The processing used to remove the fundamental frequency generally requires that two transmit pulses are used for each line of sight in the image. This reduces the frame rate by a factor of two.

Tissue Harmonic Imaging therefore improves image quality (as shown in Figures 12.14, 12.15 and 12.16). However this is achieved at the cost of a reduced depth of penetration and lower frame rate.

Summary

1. *As it travels into the patient's tissues the transmitted ultrasound pulse is progressively distorted. However, this occurs only in the central zone of the main beam where the intensity is high.*

2. *A distorted transmit pulse will give rise to distorted echoes and these have significant energy at harmonic frequencies.*

3. *In Tissue Harmonic Imaging the image is made using the second harmonic component of the echo signals, with the fundamental frequency excluded.*

4. *Undistorted echoes coming from lower intensity areas (e.g. the fringes of the main beam, sidelobes, superficial tissues) will not be seen in the image.*

5. *The result is that the image has far less beamwidth, slice thickness, sidelobe and reverberation artifacts than conventional images.*

6. *Unfortunately the frame rate is lower and the depth of penetration is reduced.*

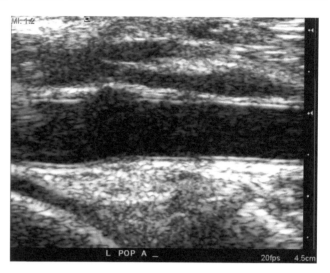

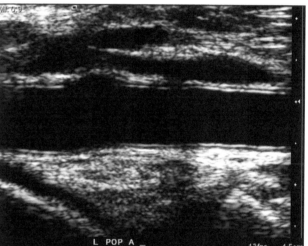

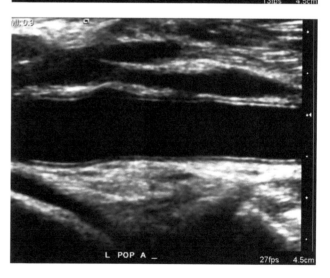

Figure 12.16 The same popliteal artery as shown in Figure 12.5. The conventional image (top) shows significant artifact echoes within the vessel lumen and a very granular speckle pattern. Harmonic imaging (centre) largely eliminates the artifacts and defines the vessel walls more clearly. Using a combination of harmonics and compound imaging (bottom) substantially smooths the speckle and displays the tissue boundaries more clearly.

Contrast harmonics

Ultrasound contrast agents increase the ultrasound reflectivity of blood by introducing very small bubbles of gas into the bloodstream. (This will be discussed in more detail in the next section.)

These bubbles behave in a distinctive way. Due to their size they resonate when exposed to ultrasound. As a result, the echoes from the bubbles are distorted and so they have a substantial amount of energy at the second harmonic frequency. This means that:

> *Echoes from contrast bubbles are significantly distorted, regardless of whether the incident ultrasound is distorted or not.*

Echoes from contrast bubbles will thus have a larger harmonic component than other echoes. It follows that using harmonic imaging in combination with contrast agents will further increase the reflectivity of blood relative to tissue.

Harmonic imaging is therefore widely used to make contrast agents more visible in the image. An example is shown in Figure 12.17. Similarly, harmonic Doppler can be used with contrast agents to increase the detectability of Doppler signals in difficult situations such as transcranial Doppler.

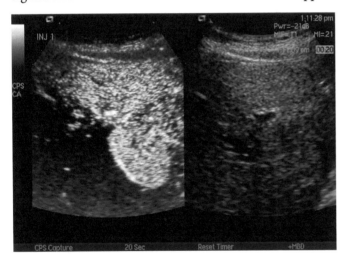

Figure 12.17 (Left) Contrast enhanced image of focal nodular hyperplasia. Note how difficult it is to see the lesion in the grey scale image on the right.

Harmonic signal processing

Figure 12.18 shows the simplest possible way to eliminate the fundamental frequency component from the echo signal.

A filter (similar to that described in chapter 4) is used to remove all but the desired range of frequencies.

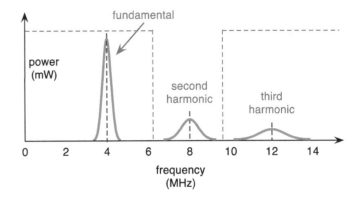

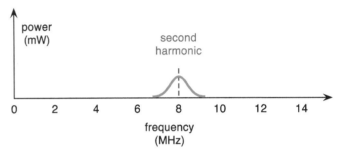

Figure 12.18 (Top) A filter (broken lines) can remove the fundamental and other unwanted frequencies from the echo signal. (Bottom) Only the second harmonic remains. This is processed to yield the image (or Doppler signal).

While this approach can work – it was used in the first generation of harmonic imaging machines – it has a major limitation. It will fail if the fundamental and second harmonic spectrums overlap (as shown in Figure 12.19), since the filter will then be unable to separate them.

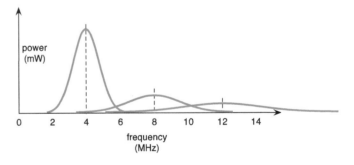

Figure 12.19 If a short transmit pulse is used (in order to achieve good image resolution) the fundamental and harmonic frequencies overlap and it is then impossible to separate them by filtering.

Unfortunately the only way to prevent overlap would be to use a relatively long transmit pulse, since this would keep the signal bandwidth relatively small. However, it would also degrade the axial resolution of the images. This limitation led to the development of "pulse inversion" harmonic signal processing. This works well even when the spectrums overlap, so there is no degradation of the axial resolution.

It does, however, require two transmit pulses for each line of sight and so the frame rate is halved. The first transmit pulse is simply the normal pulse. The machine temporarily stores the echo information from this pulse for all depths in digital format.

It then transmits a second time without moving the beam. As shown in Figure 12.20, the second transmit pulse is the inverse of the first. Again the echoes from all depths are stored. The echoes from the two transmit pulses are then added at each depth to yield a final composite echo signal.

This relatively simple process eliminates the fundamental component of the signal, retaining the second harmonic. The second harmonic signal is then processed in the usual way to produce an image (or Doppler signal).

In summary, harmonic imaging and harmonic Doppler are achieved using the pulse inversion technique to remove the fundamental frequency component from the echo signal.

When harmonic images are compared with standard images we see that:

- artifact echoes are dramatically reduced;
- ultrasound contrast agent bubbles become more echogenic relative to tissue;
- there is no compromise in spatial resolution; but
- the frame rate is halved.

Suggested activities

1. Experiment with harmonic imaging in several different application areas.
2. Acquire conventional and harmonic images of the same anatomy and compare them carefully. Note any improvements in the images and whether the spatial resolution and frame rate seem to be affected by using harmonics.

Ultrasound contrast agents

Blood is a poor scatterer of ultrasound, as shown by its lack of visibility in ultrasound images. This can be a problem at times, for example in transcranial Doppler where the ultrasound is severely attenuated as it passes through the skull. This problem spurred the development of ultrasound contrast agents with the aim of making blood more echogenic.

We have seen that gas bubbles, even very small ones, are strongly echogenic. It is no surprise therefore that ultrasound contrast agents work by introducing small gas bubbles into the bloodstream.

A considerable number of ultrasound contrast agents have been developed and several have been approved for clinical use (although this varies from country to country).

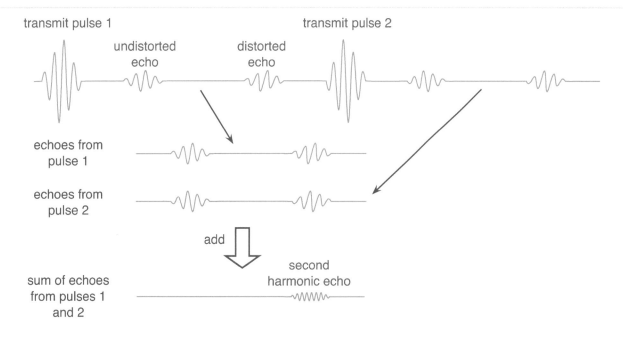

Figure 12.20 For each line of sight (beam position) the machine transmits and receives twice. The second transmit pulse is the inverse of the first. The echo signals are stored and then added to produce a composite echo signal. Undistorted echoes will be eliminated, since they are equal and opposite. The fundamental component of distorted echoes will be also be removed, leaving the second harmonic component of these echoes.

The gas in the bubbles may simply be air, carbon dioxide or something similar. However, many contrast agents use perfluorocarbon gases because these have a considerably longer lifetime in the bloodstream.

The bubbles are encapsulated using a thin shell to stabilise them. They are typically 3 – 5 microns in size (a micron is a micrometre). This allows them to pass through all the vessels in the body, including the microvasculature, without becoming trapped. (For comparison, the largest dimension of a red blood cell is 7 microns.)

Contrast agents are generally administered by intravenous injection. They increase the echogenicity of blood by a factor of 500 to 1000. The increased reflectivity lasts for a number of minutes, after which the body will remove the contrast agent from the bloodstream and excrete it. Naturally it is essential that none of the materials used should show any toxicity.

Initial applications of ultrasound contrast included:

- improving Doppler signals in difficult areas such as transcranial and renal artery Doppler;

- improving the visualisation of blood in the heart, thereby allowing more accurate outlining of the heart walls;

- visualisation of the blood supply within organs and in relation to lesions such as haematomas and malignancies.

As early adopters started to use contrast agents, other applications were developed. Some of these are based on the discovery that when the transmitted intensity (or more specifically, the MI) is increased it can destroy all the bubbles within the scan plane. An area of tissue can therefore be cleared of contrast bubbles. The ultrasound intensity can then be reduced and the bubbles will be seen returning to the area. This has been termed "perfusion imaging".

It has also been found that when the contrast bubbles are removed from the blood stream they are generally stored in the liver until they can be metabolised and excreted. Ultrasound imaging can show the bubbles where they have accumulated in the liver, particularly when harmonic imaging is used (as explained in the previous section).

Importantly, only normal functional liver tissue will take up the bubbles. Abnormal tissues in the liver (e.g. metastatic nodules) will therefore be seen as "voids" in the image (as shown in Figure 12.21).

This brief description cannot do full justice to the subject of ultrasound contrast agents.

While the clinical use of the agents varies greatly from country to country (largely due to differences in regulatory approaches), a quick look at ultrasound journals will show that a great deal of exciting work is being done with contrast agents.

One fascinating application currently in research is the use of targeted bubbles (i.e. bubbles with coatings which selectively attach to specific tissue types) to locate and/or treat diseased tissues such as thrombus and malignancies.

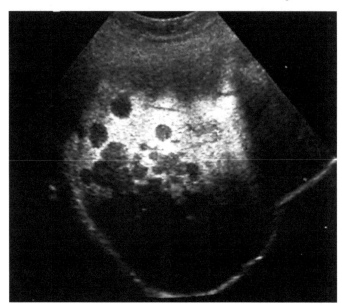

Figure 12.21 Contrast enhanced image of the liver showing the uptake of contrast bubbles in normal functional liver tissue, leaving voids where there is no normal tissue. Note the limited penetration due to the use of harmonic imaging to enhance the contrast.

3D and 4D ultrasound

Standard ultrasound imaging is inherently a two-dimensional (2D) modality, since each image represents the structures in a slice through the patient's tissues. Remember that this slice has a finite thickness, which we term the slice thickness.

Human anatomy, of course, is three dimensional (3D). It may seem that there is a mismatch between the 2D nature of standard ultrasound images and the 3D nature of the body.

However medical imaging offers highly refined ways to deal with this. In Computed Tomography (CT) and Magnetic Resonance Imaging (MRI), for example, a number of parallel image planes are acquired and displayed, and the viewer integrates them mentally to get a picture of the anatomy in three dimensions.

In ultrasound the user generally scans systematically through a region of interest, often using more than one probe orientation. Thus a kidney will be scanned by sweeping the scan plane from one end of the kidney to the other, generating a sequence of short axis views. The probe will then be rotated 90° and the scan plane will be swept from one side of the kidney to the other, generating a sequence of long axis views. The scan plane has thus been swept through the entire volume of the kidney using two different scan orientations.

The viewer can mentally integrate the information obtained to get an overall picture of the entire organ. Often measurements are required, in which case specific sections through the organ will be needed to make the measurements correctly.

While this is clearly a very successful strategy, there has long been an interest in the idea of 3D ultrasound.

This involves:

- scanning a volume of tissue automatically;
- storing the entire sequence of images acquired, along with information about the spatial position of each scan plane;
- reconstructing the resulting "volume" of echo information in a variety of image formats.

In recent years 3D ultrasound has become far more widely available and its use has exploded. For example, a quick internet search will reveal thousands of websites showing 3D fetal images. It is therefore important to understand that, as with so many of the newer ultrasound modes of operation, 3D ultrasound has significant limitations and it is therefore *complementary* to conventional 2D ultrasound.

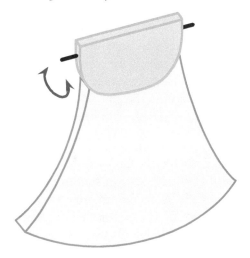

Figure 12.22 Inside a mechanical 3D probe a curved array transducer is rocked backwards and forwards by a motor. The scan plane sweeps through a volume of tissue.

How do 3D ultrasound machines sweep the scan plane through a volume of tissue?

Until recently this has been achieved by scanning the probe mechanically, as shown in Figure 12.22. Clearly this cannot be done in a fraction of a second and so it is not suited to real time 3D scanning (often called 4D).

In recent years matrix transducers have been introduced (see chapter 4 for more details).

These transducers are divided into small elements along their length (as in conventional array transducers) and also across their width. This means that electronic focussing can be applied both within the scan plane (as with conventional probes) and across the width of the transducer, substantially reducing slice thickness.

Furthermore, matrix transducers can steer the beam in both directions - within the scan plane and in the direction perpendicular to it. Thus they can sweep the scan plane rapidly through a volume of tissue, as shown in Figure 12.23, and so they are capable of producing real time 3D images.

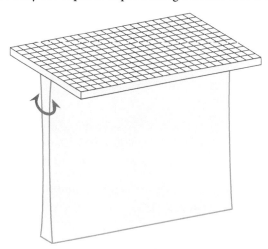

Figure 12.23 A matrix array can steer the scan plane back and forth (arrow) to scan a volume of tissues.

The images obtained as the scan plane is swept through the area of interest are stored in what might be termed a 3D image memory (see Figure 12.24).

Since the machine is creating the images it knows their spatial relationship and so we can think of there being a volume of echo information stored within the machine.

How is this turned into an image? The answer depends on the user's requirements. A range of options are available, mostly derived from techniques used in CT and MRI for displaying 3D images. Note that the process of turning a volume of data into an image on a screen is termed "rendering".

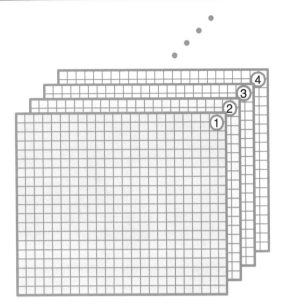

Figure 12.24 (a) As the scan plane is swept through the tissues, each image is stored in a separate image plane in the image memory. We see here the first four images.

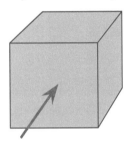

Figure 12.24 (b) The stored images can be thought of as a volume of echo data which needs to be visualised in some way. The "viewing" direction is shown by the arrow.

The simplest way to display 3D ultrasound information is for the user to define a plane through the volume of data (as shown in Figure 12.25). The machine then creates an image from the echoes that lie on this plane – you can think of it as being a "virtual" scan plane.

This is often called "reslicing" the image data.

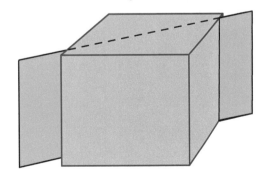

Figure 12.25 A plane (positioned by the user) slices through the volume of echo data. An image is created using the echo data intersected by the plane.

Benefits of reslicing include:

- you can select the correct plane to visualise structures of interest and to make measurements;
- you can obtain a virtual scan plane with an orientation that could not be obtained with conventional scanning.

A major limitation of 3D ultrasound (at present) is the relatively poor resolution in the slice thickness direction. When the image data is resliced the slice thickness significantly degrades image quality. Matrix transducers should significantly improve this aspect of 3D ultrasound.

Another simple way to display the volume of image data is to use "volume rendering", as shown in Figure 12.26. Unfortunately this is not generally useful in ultrasound because the resulting image is too cluttered with echoes.

However, there are two related techniques which can be very effective in specific situations.

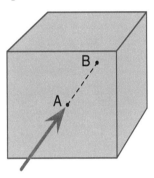

Figure 12.26 In volume rendering all of the echoes along the line from A to B are combined and displayed at the point A. Thus all the echoes in the entire volume are combined to form a 2D image.

The first of these is termed "maximum projection". Referring again to Figure 12.26, all the echoes along the line from A to B are examined and the *strongest* echo is selected and displayed at the point A. Thus the image is made up of the strongest echoes along each sight line.

This can be very effective where there is a well defined source of strong echoes such as the fetal skeleton. Another popular application of this method is in vascular ultrasound. An image can be made by maximum projection using colour Doppler and ignoring the grey scale information. (Often power mode colour Doppler is used due to its more consistent appearance.)

Maximum projection imaging, in conjunction with harmonics, is also used to visualise the build-up of contrast bubbles in an organ such as the kidney.

This is even more effective when the image is allowed to build up over a period of a few seconds.

The other useful technique related to volume rendering is "surface rendering". Again the machine looks at each viewing line into the volume of echo data (as shown in Figure 12.26). However in this case it would select the first significant echo along the line AB and display it at the point A.

Moreover, since the machine knows the depth of each displayed echo, it can artificially "light" the image from one side to emphasise curved surfaces.

Surface rendering can produce very effective views of structures such as the fetal face or the interior surfaces of the heart. These images can be a valuable aid for communicating findings to non-imaging specialists (e.g. paediatric surgeons) and to patients and their families.

With both maximum projection and surface rendering, a further improvement can be obtained if a number of images are produced, each looking at the data from a slightly different viewing angle.

These can be assembled into a movie loop. When it is played, the reconstructed anatomy rotates back and forth. This can significantly improve the viewer's appreciation of the relative depth of different structures in the image.

A completely different approach is the use of "orthogonal plane" viewing of the volume of data.

Three slices are taken through the image, each perpendicular to the others as shown in Figure 12.27 ("orthogonal" simply means at right angles). The three images are all displayed on the screen. The user can then manipulate their position in the anatomy, moving them anywhere within the volume of data.

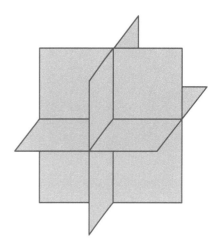

Figure 12.27 The most comprehensive display of 3D ultrasound shows three images simultaneously. The images are "orthogonal", meaning that they are perpendicular to one another, as shown here.

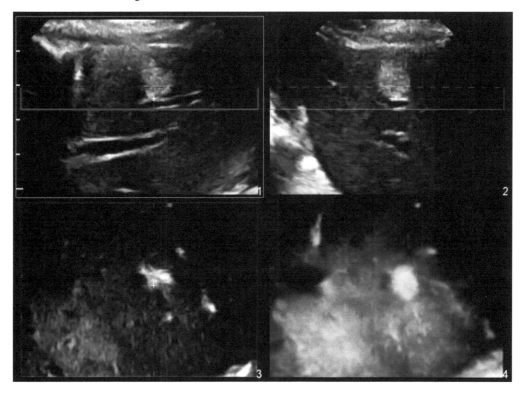

Figure 12.28 An echogenic liver mass imaged using a 9000+ element matrix array transducer. The three orthogonal grey scale images are in sagittal, transverse and coronal planes. The bottom right image is a volume rendering of the mass and the surrounding liver tissue.

This style of display has been used since the early days of 3D imaging. It is very comprehensive but rather difficult to understand on first viewing. It is widely used with invasive imaging, for example in gynaecology and prostate imaging.

A variant, biplane imaging, is also commonly used with transoesophageal imaging of the heart. Figure 12.28 is a clinical 3D image using a combination of the orthogonal plane approach and volume rendering.

The term "4D ultrasound" is often used to describe real time 3D images. Two approaches can be taken to producing real time 3D:

- a series of 3D images is acquired over a period of many seconds; the patient's electrocardiogram is also recorded, enabling the machine to assemble the images into a video loop showing a "representative" heart cycle;
- with matrix transducers it is possible to sweep the scan plane back and forth through a limited volume of tissue sufficiently quickly that genuine real time 3D images (using surface rendering, for example) can be displayed "live".

In summary, 3D and 4D ultrasound are now part of regular clinical ultrasound practice, particularly in fetal scanning. A variety of different methods for viewing the 3D information are available, the most useful being reslicing, surface rendering, maximum projection and orthogonal plane viewing.

Unfortunately the relatively poor slice thickness of conventional array transducers is still a major limitation. However, the advent of matrix transducers promises to improve slice thickness and enable real time 3D imaging.

Extended field of view

This function allows the field of view of an ultrasound image to be extended by moving the probe over the patient's skin and building up the width of the image as shown in Figure 12.29.

As each new image is generated by the machine it is "stitched" onto the displayed image in the correct location. This is almost identical to the panoramic imaging function often available with digital cameras; some ultrasound equipment manufacturers even call it "panoramic imaging".

With good technique the quality of the extended field of view image is similar to a standard image (see Figure 12.30).

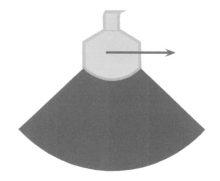

Figure 12.29 (a) The user moves the probe over the patient's skin surface, ensuring that the orientation of the scan plane is maintained.

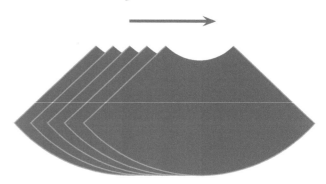

Figure 12.29 (b) Each new image is added to the existing image in the correct location, extending the field of view.

On the other hand, Figure 12.31 shows a typical artifact caused by inaccurate "stitching" of the images. Commonly this occurs when the user inadvertently tilts the probe while moving it, or when the patient moves during the image acquisition.

The extended field of view function can be useful. In general it is used quite selectively, mainly to obtain a "record" image of an examination with a large field of view.

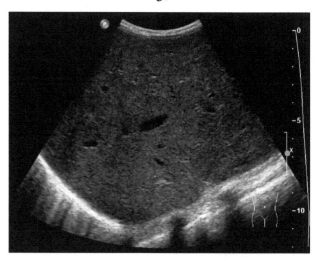

Figure 12.30 (a) Standard image of a liver.

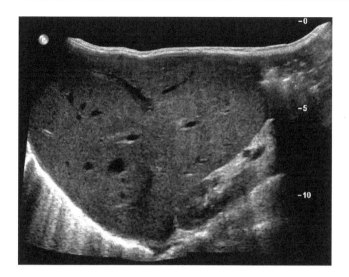

Figure 12.30 (b) Extended field of view image of the liver.

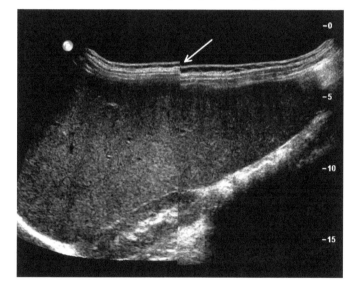

Figure 12.31 The discontinuity in this image (arrow) has been caused by a failure to correctly stitch the images together at one point.

Image optimisation

A number of machines feature a control which allows the user to nominate an area in the image which they want the machine to "optimise".

The image in the vicinity of this area of interest is analysed and the machine then adjusts the gain, TGC, dynamic range etc to attempt to make the image quality in this area as good as possible.

Naturally the machine has its own way of determining what an "optimum" image is, and it may or may not coincide with human judgement of image quality.

This can be a useful function at times to get the machine's settings close to optimum, with the user then fine-tuning them for best results.

Image manipulation

Ultrasound machines have exploited the rapid development of computer technology in many ways. An example is this function which is available on a number of machines. The machine applies a modest amount of post-processing manipulation of the ultrasound image to improve its appearance and (it is hoped) to improve its diagnostic value. This Photoshop-style manipulation generally includes the detection and smoothing of speckle and enhancement of boundaries.

Elastography

In clinical medicine extensive use is made of palpation. This is because many disease processes alter the physical properties of tissue. Diseased tissues are often harder than normal tissues, for example.

In recent years, ultrasonic techniques have been developed for assessing the elasticity of tissue (i.e. its "stiffness"), and this function is now available in a number of current ultrasound machines. Of particular interest is its use in assessing tissues which are too deep in the body to be palpated manually.

A force is applied to the tissues, either by manually pushing on the probe or by creating an ultrasonic shock wave which travels through the tissues. The movement of the tissues is then detected from a series of ultrasound images and analysed. Stiffer areas of tissue will compress less than soft tissue and they can therefore be highlighted in the image.

Potential applications for this technology include the detection of masses in the breast and liver.

Suggested activities

1. Try to get access to a machine with one or more of the technologies above and experiment with them.

2. Observe how they are used in clinical practice, and how the information that they provide can contribute to the diagnostic process.

Summary

This brings us to the end of our journey through the physics and technology of diagnostic ultrasound. You should now feel confident that you can use ultrasound equipment safely and effectively.

You should also have a good foundation for the continued development of your clinical skills and knowledge.

Since ultrasound technology and applications are constantly changing and increasing in their sophistication, you are now condemned to a lifetime of keeping up to date!

There are many ways to do this:

- read journals, newsletters, websites;
- participate in seminars, workshops and professional conferences;
- visit the equipment exhibition and information sessions often found at professional conferences;
- read material on manufacturers' websites and their "white papers" which they publish to explain new technology;
- participate in courses and continuing education sessions.

Take advantage of these resources and keep your knowledge current. If you have grasped the material in this book, you should find this at least manageable and perhaps even enjoyable!

Answers to mathematical exercises

Chapter 1 exercises

1. $y = \dfrac{x}{7}$

2. $y = x - 7$

3. $y = \dfrac{3x + 9}{2}$

4. $y = \dfrac{x + 5}{z - 5}$

5. 2 (most easily calculated by taking 3 from 3 first, leaving the 2).

6. 2 (you can multiply (3×2) first then divide by 3, or divide 2 by 3 then multiply by 3, or best of all recognise that $(3 \div 3)$ gives 1 leaving just 2).

7. 2.5 (make sure you calculate $(8 - 3)$ first; also note that you must calculate $(6 + 2)$ before dividing by it).

8. 11.67 (divide top and bottom by 8 first, then calculate).

9. 5.6 cm (or 56 mm) (convert 16 mm to 1.6 cm or 4 cm to 40 mm first).

10. 25.04 m^2 (convert 20 cm to 0.2 m first).

11. 7.7×10^6 (convert to 1.54×10^3 m/sec and 2×10^{-4} m/sec first).

12. 10^5.

13. 10.

14. 10^{-1}.

15. 2.43×10^5.

16. 4.35×10^{-4}.

17. $(2.82 \times 10^3) \times (3.2 \times 10^{-3}) = (2.82 \times 3.2) = 9.024$.

18. 8.979×10^2.

19. $\log 20 = 1.3$; $(\log 2 + \log 10 = 0.3 + 1 = 1.3)$.

20. $\log (50 \div 25) = \log 2 = 0.3$; $(\log 50 - \log 25 = 1.7 - 1.4 = 0.3)$.

21. sin: 0, 0.5, 0.707, 0.866, 1; cos: 1, 0.866, 0.707, 0.5, 0.

22. $\sin^{-1}$: 0°, 30°, 45°, 90°; $\cos^{-1}$: 90°, 60°, 45°, 0°.

23. 61.4 dB.

24. 5×10^5; $(10 \log (\text{atten}) = 57$ and so $\log (\text{atten}) = 57/10 = 5.7$ and therefore atten $= 10^{5.7} = 5 \times 10^5)$.

Page 11

2   32, 27, 16, 11, 8, 5.3 cm

Page 14

1   96%, 96%

2   0.001%

3   R = 0.83%, T = 99.17%, R + T = 100%

Page 16

2   65°

Page 19

1 (a)   5

3   0.25 μsec

Page 21

1 (a)   104 μsec

1 (b)   20.8 msec

1 (c)   48 Hz

1 (d) $(FR \times P \times N) = 76{,}800$

Page 32

3   3.0 mm

Page 37

1   0.94 mm

2   3.8 mm

3   16.6 msec, 60 Hz

Page 76

2   1.30 kHz

3   1.41 kHz, 8.9%

Index

Lightning Source UK Ltd
Milton Keynes UK
UKHW050946301019
352562UK00003B/13/P